Gastrointestinal Radiology

Companion

Imaging Fundamentals

Gastrointestinal Radiology
Companion

Imaging Fundamentals

Ronald L. Eisenberg, M.D., J.D.

Chairman of Radiology
Alameda County Medical Center
Oakland, California

Clinical Professor of Radiology
University of California at San Francisco
University of California at Davis

LIPPINCOTT WILLIAMS & WILKINS
A **Wolters Kluwer** Company
Philadelphia • Baltimore • New York • London
Buenos Aires • Hong Kong • Sydney • Tokyo

Acquisitions Editor: James Ryan
Developmental Editor: Carol Field
Manufacturing Manager: Dennis Teston
Production Manager: Cassie Moore
Production Editor: Rita Madrigal
Cover Designer: Pinho Graphic Design
Indexer: Lisa Mulleneaux
Compositor: Lippincott Williams & Wilkins Desktop Division
Printer: Maple Press

Printed in the United States of America

9 8 7 6 5 4 3 2 1

Library of Congress Cataloging-in-Publication Data
Eisenberg, Ronald L.
    Gastrointestinal radiology companion : imaging fundamentals /
    Ronald L. Eisenberg.
        p.   cm.
    Includes bibliographical references and index.
    ISBN 0-7817-1946-1
    1. Gastrointestinal system—Radiography.   2. Gastrointestinal system—
Radiography—Atlases.   I. Eisenberg, Ronald L. Gastrointestinal radiology.   II. Title.
    [DNLM: 1. Gastrointestinal Diseases—radiography outlines.
2. Gastrointestinal Diseases—radiography atlases.   WI 141E36g 1996
Suppl. 1998]
    RC804.R6E374 1998
    616.3'07572—dc21
    DNLM/DLC
for Library of Congress   98-29513
                                                                          CIP

To Zina, Avlana, and Cherina

CONTENTS

Part E: Colon

Part F: Gallbladder and Biliary Tree

Part G: Liver

Part H: Pancreas

Part I: Spleen

Part J: Appendix, Mesentery, Peritoneal Cavity

Part K: Miscellaneous

PREFACE

This companion has been designed to provide a brief overview of the broad spectrum of gastrointestinal radiology. It is intended as a convenient and practical source of information rather than as a complete and comprehensive reference work. For each of 250 conditions, there is a short series of "Key Facts" detailing the major clinical and imaging findings. This is followed by one or more illustrations of the characteristic radiographic appearance, combining conventional radiology and barium studies with ultrasound and computed tomography. "Suggested Reading" sections refer the interested reader to a journal article or book that discusses each subject in more detail.

This book can be used as a handy guide for both radiology residents and practicing radiologists performing gastrointestinal imaging studies. It is also valuable for medical students and referring clinicians, especially in studying for the gastrointestinal imaging portions of their board examinations.

Ronald L. Eisenberg, M.D., J.D.

Gastrointestinal Radiology

Companion

Imaging Fundamentals

Part A
ESOPHAGUS

1 Motility Disorders

Cricopharyngeal Achalasia

KEY FACTS

- Failure of pharyngeal peristalsis to coordinate with relaxation of the upper esophageal sphincter (due to some interference with complex neuromuscular activity in this region)
- Hemispherical or horizontal, shelf-like protrusion on the posterior aspect of the esophagus at approximately the C5-C6 level
- Usually asymptomatic, but can result in dysphagia by obstructing the passage of a swallowed bolus
- In severe disease, can cause aspiration and pneumonia
- May lead to the development of a Zenker's diverticulum

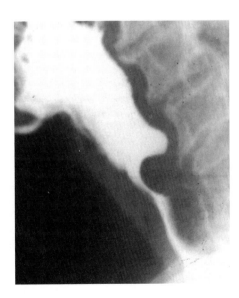

FIGURE 1-1
Cricopharyngeal achalasia. Severe posterior impression causing narrowing of the esophageal lumen.

Suggested Reading
Torres WE, Clements JL, Austin GE, et al. Cricopharyngeal muscle hypertrophy: radiological-anatomic correlation. *AJR* 1984;141:927.

Achalasia

KEY FACTS

- Functional obstruction of the distal esophagus with proximal dilatation, caused by incomplete relaxation of the lower esophageal sphincter
- Paucity or absence of ganglion cells in the myenteric plexuses (Auerbach's) of the distal esophageal wall
- Slowly progressive dysphagia developing over many months or years
- Characteristic imaging findings include:
  a. Dilatation and tortuousity of the esophagus causing a widened mediastinum (often with an air-fluid level) primarily on the right side adjacent to the cardiac shadow
  b. Multiple uncoordinated tertiary contractions
  c. Smooth tapered, conical narrowing of the distal esophagus (beak sign)
  d. Small spurts of barium entering the stomach on erect films (jet effect)
  e. Small or absent gastric air bubble
- Must be distinguished from pseudo-achalasia due to invasion of the distal esophagus by carcinoma of the gastric cardia (older age group, >50; shorter duration of symptoms, <6 months)

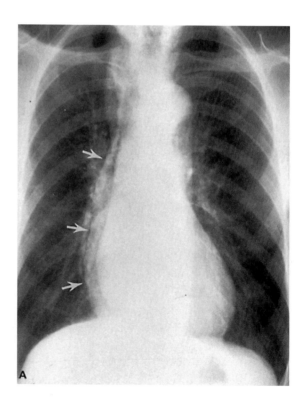

FIGURE 1-2

Achalasia. The margin of the dilated, tortuous esophagus *(arrows)* parallels the right border of the heart.

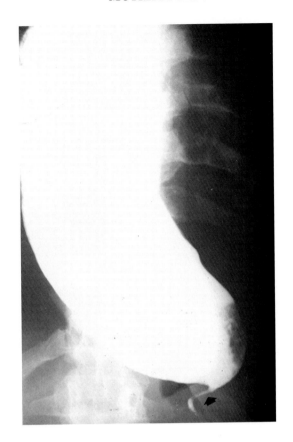

F I G U R E   1 - 3

Achalasia. Massive dilatation of the esophagus proximal to a tight narrowing of the distal esophagus *(arrow)*.

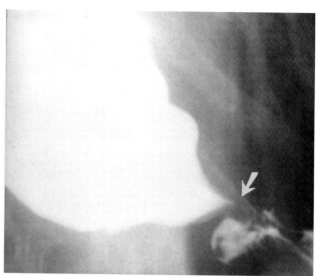

A

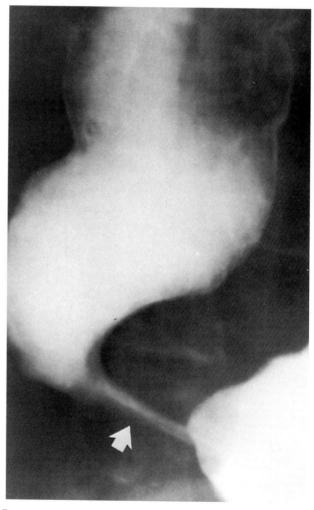

B

FIGURE 1-4
Achalasia. **A:** Beak sign
(arrow). **B:** Jet effect.

Suggested Readings

Agha FP. Secondary neoplasms of the esophagus. *Gastrointest Radiol* 1987;12:187.
Zboralske FF, Dodds WJ. Roentgenographic diagnosis of primary disorders of esophageal
    motility. *Radiol Clin North Am* 1969;7:147.

Chagas Disease

KEY FACTS

- Destruction of the myenteric plexuses by the protozoan *Trypanosome cruzi*
- Develops from the bite of an infected reduviid bug (armadillo is the chief host)
- Radiographic pattern identical to achalasia
- Also causes dilatation of small bowel loops, megacolon with chronic constipation, ureteral dilatation, and myocarditis

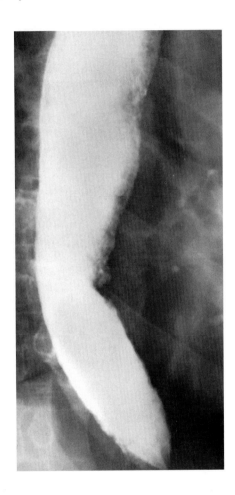

FIGURE 1-5
Chagas disease. Esophageal dilatation and aperistalsis with a large amount of residual food.

Suggested Reading

Reeder MM, Hamilton LC. Radiologic diagnosis of tropical diseases of the gastrointestinal tract. *Radiol Clin North Am* 1969;7:57.

Scleroderma

KEY FACTS

- Progressive atrophy of smooth muscle with replacement by fibrosis
- Involves the esophagus in about 80% of cases, sometimes before the characteristic skin changes become evident
- Often asymptomatic, though the patient may be required to eat or drink in a sitting or erect position
- Normal stripping wave in the upper third of the esophagus (striated muscle) with dilated, atonic esophagus from the aortic arch down (smooth muscle)
- High incidence of gastroesophageal reflux through a patulous lower esophageal sphincter, leading to peptic esophagitis and stricture formation
- In the upright position, barium flows rapidly into the stomach (unlike the jet effect in achalasia)

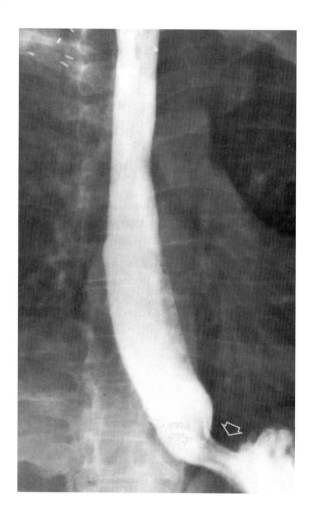

FIGURE 1-6
Scleroderma. The esophagus is dilated and atonic, and the esophagogastric junction is patulous *(arrow)*.

Suggested Reading
Margulis AR, Koehler RE. Radiologic diagnosis of disordered esophageal motility: a unified physiologic approach. *Radiol Clin North Am* 1976;14:429.

Diffuse Esophageal Spasm

KEY FACTS

- Clinical triad of massive uncoordinated esophageal contractions, chest pain, and increased intramural pressure
- Symptoms are frequently caused or aggravated by eating, but can occur spontaneously and even awaken the patient at night
- Tertiary contractions of abnormally high amplitude that can obliterate the lumen (pronounced corkscrew pattern)

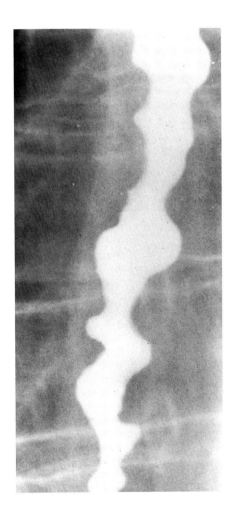

FIGURE 1-7
Diffuse esophageal spasm. High-amplitude contractions irregularly narrow the lumen of the esophagus.

Suggested Reading

Chen YM, Ott DJ, Hewson EG, et al. Diffuse esophageal spasm: radiographic and manometric correlation. *Radiology* 1989;170:807.

Presbyesophagus

KEY FACTS

- Defect in primary peristalsis with nonpropulsive tertiary contractions
- Associated with aging (especially age >70 years)
- May result from a minor cerebrovascular accident affecting the central nuclei
- Usually asymptomatic, but can cause moderate dysphagia

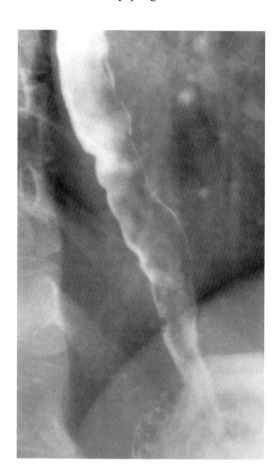

FIGURE 1-8
Presbyesophagus. Diffuse tertiary contractions.

Suggested Reading
Seaman WB. Pathophysiology of the esophagus. *Semin Roentgenol* 1981;16:214.

2 Extrinsic Impressions on Cervical Portion

Cricopharyngeus Muscle

KEY FACTS

- Posterior impression at the C5-C6 level
- Caused by failure of the cricopharyngeus muscle to relax

Suggested Reading
Ekberg O, Nylander G. Dysfunction of the cricopharyngeal muscle. *Radiology* 1982;143:481.

Pharyngeal Venous Plexus

KEY FACTS

- Anterior impression at the C6 level (appearance varies from swallow to swallow)
- Caused by prolapse of lax mucosal folds over the rich central submucosal pharyngeal venous plexus (considered a normal finding)

Esophageal Web

KEY FACTS

- Smooth, thin lucent band (covered by squamous epithelium) arising from the anterior wall of the esophagus near the pharyngoesophageal junction
- Usually asymptomatic and an incidental finding
- Rarely multiple or distal

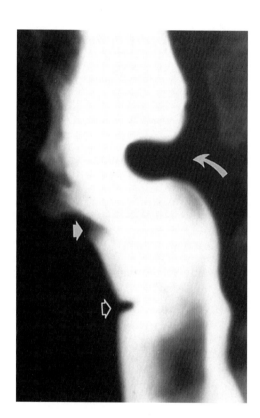

FIGURE 2-1

Three normal extrinsic impressions on the cervical esophagus. Cricopharyngeus muscle *(curved arrow)*, pharyngeal venous plexus (short closed arrow), and esophageal web *(short open arrow)*. (From Clements JL, Cox GW, Torres WE, et al. Cervical esophageal webs: a roentgen-anatomic correlation. *AJR* 1974;121:221, with permission.)

Suggested Reading

Clements JL, Cox GW, Torres WE, et al. Cervical esophageal webs: a roentgen-anatomic correlation. *AJR* 1974;121:221.

Anterior Marginal Osteophyte

KEY FACTS

- Smooth, regular indentation of the posterior wall at the level of an intervertebral disk space
- Usually asymptomatic, but may produce pain or difficulty in swallowing [especially with profuse osteophytosis and diffuse idiopathic skeletal hyperostosis (DISH)]

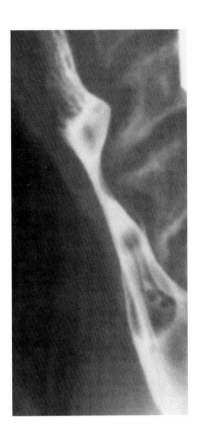

FIGURE 2-2
Anterior marginal osteophyte. Smooth, regular indentation on the posterior wall at the level of an intervertebral disk space.

Suggested Reading

Resnick D, Shaul SR, Robbins JM. Diffuse idiopathic skeletal hyperostosis (DISH). Forrestier's disease with extraspinal manifestations. *Radiology* 1975;115:513.

Thyroid Enlargement or Mass

KEY FACTS

- Smooth impression on and displacement of the lateral wall of the esophagus (usually with parallel effects on the trachea)
- Caused by localized or generalized hypertrophy of the gland, inflammatory disease, or thyroid malignancy

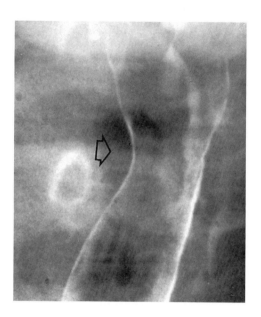

FIGURE 2-3
Thyroid enlargement. Smooth impression *(arrow)* on the cervical esophagus.

3 Inflammatory Disease

Reflux Esophagitis

KEY FACTS

- Esophageal inflammation secondary to reflux of acid-peptic contents from the stomach
- Increased incidence with hiatal hernia, repeated vomiting, prolonged nasogastric intubation, scleroderma, and late pregnancy
- Radiographic findings include diffuse superficial or deep erosions with nodular thickening of mucosal folds
- May be associated with a disorder of esophageal motility and fine transverse folds (feline esophagus)
- Fibrotic healing results in an asymmetric, often irregular, stricture of the distal esophagus that usually extends to the cardioesophageal junction (unlike Barrett's stricture, in which a variable length of normal-appearing esophagus separates the stricture from the cardioesophageal junction)

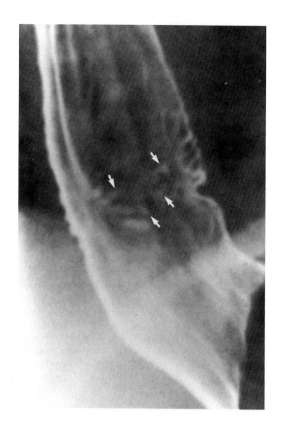

FIGURE 3-1

Reflux esophagitis. Multiple tiny ulcers *(arrows)* are seen en face in the distal esophagus near the gastroesophageal junction. Note the radiating folds and puckering of the adjacent esophageal wall. (From Gore RM, Levine MS, Laufer I, eds. *Textbook of gastrointestinal radiology.* Philadelphia: WB Saunders, 1994, with permission.)

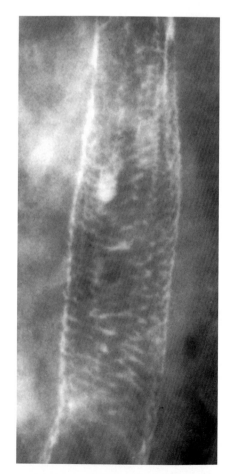

FIGURE 3-2

Reflux esophagitis. Prominent transverse esophageal folds (feline esophagus). (From Gohel VK, Edell S, Laufer I, et al. Transverse folds in the human esophagus. *Radiology* 1978;128:303, with permission.)

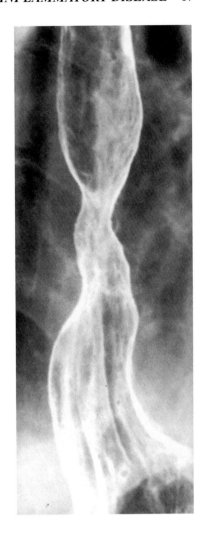

FIGURE 3-3

Reflux esophagitis. Smooth narrowing of the distal esophagus extends to the level of the hiatal hernia.

Suggested Reading

Laufer I. Radiology of esophagitis. *Radiol Clin North Am* 1982;20:687.

Barrett's Esophagus

KEY FACTS

- Replacement of normal stratified squamous lining of the lower esophagus by columnar epithelium similar to that of the stomach
- Often associated with hiatal hernia and reflux, though the ulcer is generally separated from the hernia by a variable length of normal-appearing esophagus
- Large, deep ulceration typically involves the region of the squamocolumnar junction
- Radionuclide technetium scanning shows isotope uptake in the gastric type of mucosa in the distal esophagus
- Short and tight, though smooth, post-inflammatory stricture often develops in the midesophagus at the squamocolumnar junction
- High propensity (up to 15%) for developing adenocarcinoma in the columnar-lined portion of the esophagus

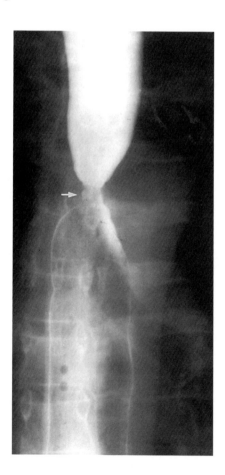

FIGURE 3-4

Barrett's esophagus. Small ulcer *(arrow)* that is separated from the hiatal hernia sac by several centimeters of normal-appearing esophagus.

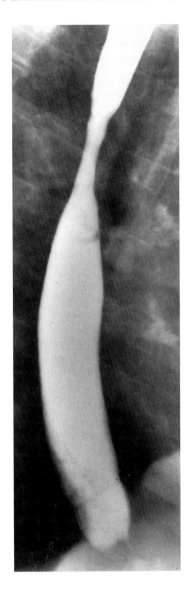

FIGURE 3-5

Barrett's esophagus. Smooth stricture in the upper thoracic esophagus. Note that the distal esophagus appears normal.

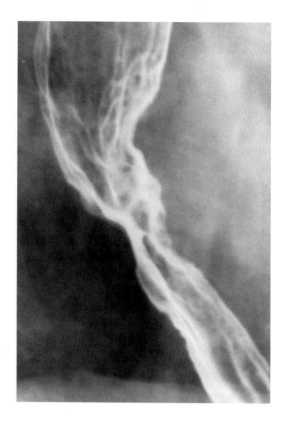

FIGURE 3-6
Adenocarcinoma in Barrett's esophagus.
Irregular, infiltrating stricture. (From
Levine MS, Caroline D, Thompson JJ, et
al. Adenocarcinoma of the esophagus:
relationship to Barrett's esophagus.
Radiology 1984;150:305, with
permission.)

Suggested Reading

Levine MS, Caroline D, Thompson JJ, et al. Adenocarcinoma of the esophagus: relationship
to Barrett's esophagus. *Radiology* 1984;150:305.

Infectious Esophagitis

KEY FACT

- Increasingly common because of the use of steroid and cytotoxic drugs, and the increasing incidence of acquired immunodeficiency syndrome (AIDS)

CANDIDA ESOPHAGITIS

KEY FACTS

- Most common infectious disease of the esophagus
- Usually develops in patients with chronic debilitating diseases or on immunosuppressive therapy
- More than 75% of patients with AIDS suffer from oroesophageal candidiasis during the course of the disease (development of dysphagia and retrosternal pain in immunosuppressed patients strongly suggests the diagnosis)
- Multiple ulcerations of various sizes that frequently involve the entire thoracic esophagus
- Irregular, nodular, plaque-like mucosal pattern with marginal serrations ("shaggy" appearance)
- Disordered esophageal motility (dilated, atonic esophagus) is often an early finding

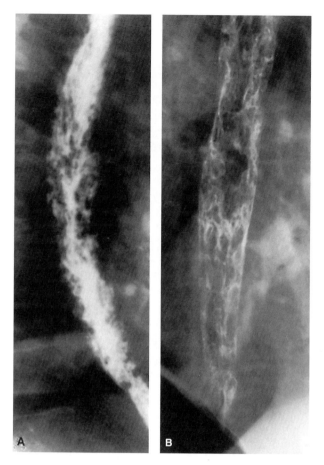

FIGURE 3-7   *Candida* esophagitis. **A:** Grossly irregular contour producing a shaggy appearance. **B:** Nodular plaque formation. (From Gore RM, Levine MS, Laufer I, eds. *Textbook of gastrointestinal radiology.* Philadelphia: WB Saunders, 1994, with permission.)

Suggested Reading

Levine MS, Woldenberg R, Herlinger H, et al. Opportunistic esophagitis in AIDS: radiographic diagnosis. *Radiology* 1987;165:815.

HERPES ESOPHAGITIS

KEY FACTS

- Self-limited viral inflammation that predominantly affects patients with disseminated malignancy or abnormal immune systems
- Radiographic appearance similar to candidiasis, though the background mucosa is often otherwise normal

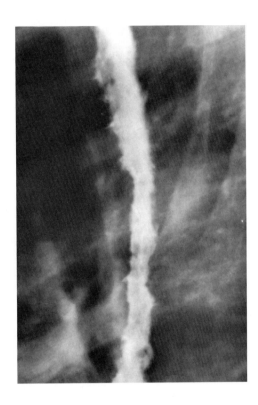

FIGURE 3-8
Herpes esophagitis. Diffuse irregularity and ulceration that is indistinguishable from *Candida* esophagitis.

Suggested Reading
Levine MS, Laufer I, Kressel HY, et al. Herpes esophagitis. *AJR* 1981;136:863.

CYTOMEGALOVIRUS ESOPHAGITIS

KEY FACTS

- Most frequently develops in patients with AIDS, disseminated malignancy, or organ transplantation
- Diffuse or segmental ulcerating process that primarily affects the distal half of the esophagus (and may extend into the gastric fundus)
- Giant flat ulcer, often with a thin rim of edematous mucosa, is highly suggestive

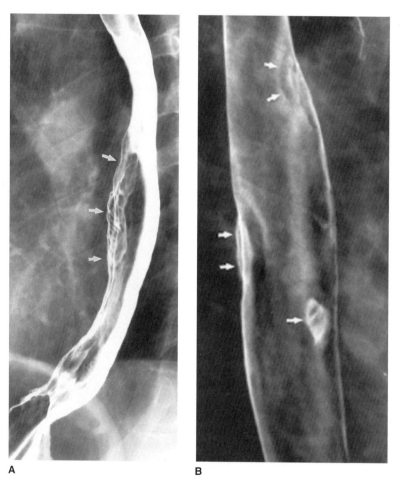

A   B

FIGURE 3-9   Cytomegalovirus esophagitis. **A:** Four discrete ulcers *(arrows).*
B: Inflammatory mucosal changes involving a short segment of the
distal esophagus *(arrows).* (From Balthazar EJ, Megibow AJ, Hulnick
DH. Cytomegalovirus esophagitis and gastritis in AIDS. *AJR* 1985;144:
1201, with permission.)

Suggested Reading
Balthazar EJ, Megibow AJ, Hulnick DH. Cytomegalovirus esophagitis and gastritis in AIDS.
   AJR 1985;144:1201.

HUMAN IMMUNODEFICIENCY VIRUS (HIV) ESOPHAGITIS

KEY FACTS

- Diagnosis of exclusion when repeated brushings, biopsies, and cultures fail to detect any signs of the usual viral or fungal organisms that are associated with opportunistic esophagitis in HIV-positive patients
- Typically giant, relatively flat, ovoid or irregular ulcers that generally involve the middle third of the esophagus (identical appearance to cytomegalovirus)

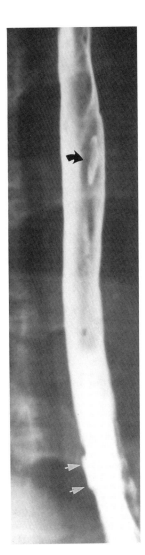

FIGURE 3-10

HIV-related ulcers. Long ovoid lesion seen en face in the upper esophagus *(black arrow)*. Note the more distal lesion *(white arrows)* seen in profile.

Suggested Reading
Levine MS, Woldenberg R, Herlinger H, et al. Opportunistic esophagitis in AIDS: radiographic diagnosis. *Radiology* 1987;165:815.

Corrosive Esophagitis

KEY FACTS

- Most severe corrosive injuries are caused by alkalis (lye, dishwashing detergents, washing soda)
- Diffuse superficial or deep ulceration involving a long portion of the distal esophagus
- Fibrotic healing results in a long esophageal stricture that extends down to the cardioesophageal junction

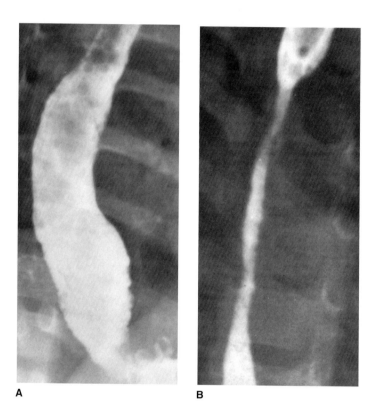

A   B

FIGURE 3-11   Corrosive esophagitis. **A:** Dilated, boggy esophagus with ulceration 8 days after the ingestion of a caustic agent. **B:** Esophagram performed 3 months later shows extensive stricture formation.

Suggested Reading
Franken EA. Caustic damage of the gastrointestinal tract: roentgen features. *AJR* 1973;118: 77.

Radiation Esophagitis

KEY FACTS

- Develops in patients with a history of radiation therapy >4,500 rads (45 Gy)
- Less than half that radiation dose produces similar changes if the patient has received simultaneous or sequential Adriamycin
- Acutely, multiple shallow or deep ulcerations of various size in the treatment field
- Radiographic appearance is indistinguishable from candidal esophagitis (far more common condition in patients undergoing chemotherapy and radiation therapy for malignant disease)
- Fibrotic healing produces a smooth tapered stricture

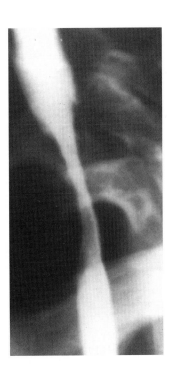

FIGURE 3-12
Radiation-induced stricture. Tapered margins and smooth mucosal surface produce a benign appearance in this stricture that developed after mediastinal radiation therapy.

Suggested Reading
Boal DKB, Newburger PE, Teel RL. Esophagitis induced by combined radiation and Adriamycin. *AJR* 1979;132:567.

4 Neoplasms

Esophageal Leiomyoma

KEY FACTS

- Most common benign esophageal neoplasm (most frequently in lower third)
- Usually asymptomatic and rarely ulcerates, bleeds, or undergoes malignant transformation
- Occasionally contains pathognomonic amorphous calcification
- Typically appears as a smooth, rounded intramural filling defect that is sharply demarcated from the adjacent esophageal wall

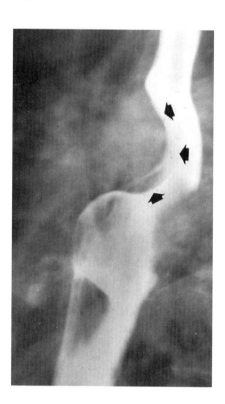

FIGURE 4-1
Leiomyoma. Smooth, rounded intramural defect in the barium column *(arrows).*

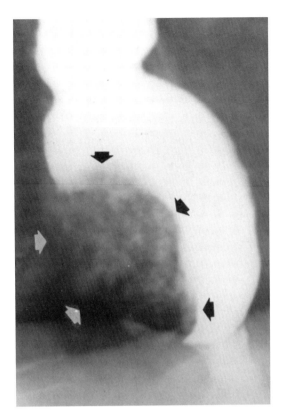

FIGURE 4-2

Leiomyoma. Amorphous calcifications *(arrows)* within a smoothly lobulated intramural tumor of the distal esophagus. (From Ghahremani GG, Meyers MA, Port RB. Calcified primary tumors of the gastrointestinal tract. *Gastrointest Radiol* 1978;2:331, with permission.)

Suggested Reading

Ghahremani GG, Meyers MA, Port RB. Calcified primary tumors of the gastrointestinal tract. *Gastrointest Radiol* 1978;2:331.

Esophageal Carcinoma

KEY FACTS

- Major cause of dysphagia in patients >40 years of age (progressive difficulty swallowing in this age group must be considered to be esophageal cancer until proven otherwise)
- Close association with drinking and smoking and with head and neck carcinomas
- Predisposing factors include Barrett's esophagus, achalasia, lye stricture, tylosis
- Symptoms tend to appear late in the course of disease, so that the tumor is often at an advanced stage when first detected radiographically
- Lack of a serosal covering on the esophagus permits the tumor to spread rapidly by direct invasion into adjacent tissues, contributing to the dismal prognosis
- Major radiographic appearances:
  a. flat plaque-like lesion on one wall of the esophagus
  b. encircling mass with irregular luminal narrowing and overhanging margins
  c. polypoid (often fungating) filling defect
  d. large ulcer niche within a bulging mass
- CT (and potentially MRI) can accurately stage the tumor preoperatively by identifying:
  a. invasion of adjacent tissues (tracheobronchial tree, aorta, pericardium)
  b. mediastinal adenopathy
  c. metastases to the liver and abdominal lymph nodes

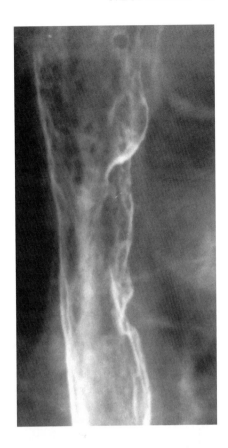

FIGURE 4-3

Early esophageal carcinoma. Irregular mass involves the left wall of the esophagus.

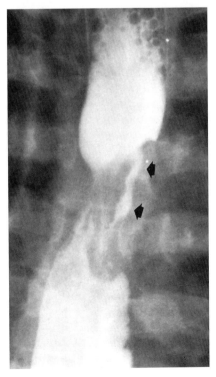

FIGURE 4-4

Carcinoma of the esophagus. Long ulceration *(arrows)* within a large rigid lesion with overhanging margins.

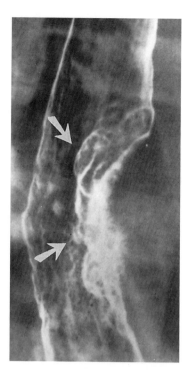

FIGURE 4-5
Carcinoma of the esophagus. Localized polypoid mass with ulceration *(arrows)*.

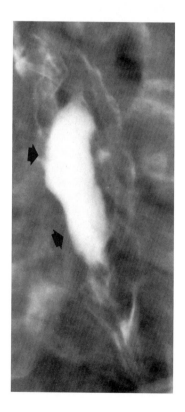

FIGURE 4-6
Primary ulcerative carcinoma. Large meniscoid ulceration *(arrows)* surrounded by a tumor mass.

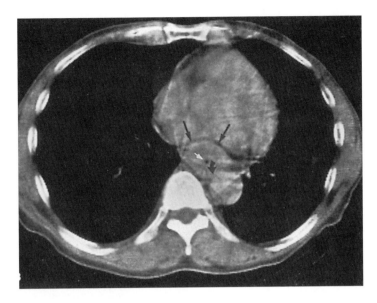

FIGURE 4-7 Carcinoma of the esophagus. CT scan shows the circumferential mass of a bulky carcinoma *(straight black arrows)* filling the lumen *(white arrow)*. Obliteration of the fat plane adjacent to the aorta *(curved arrow)* indicates mediastinal invasion.

Suggested Reading

Gore RM, Levine MS, Laufer I, eds. *Textbook of gastrointestinal imaging.* Philadelphia: WB Saunders, 1994.

Direct Spread to the Distal Esophagus from Gastric Carcinoma

KEY FACTS

- About 10% to 15% of adenocarcinomas of the stomach (2% to 10% of lymphomas) arising near the cardia invade the lower esophagus at an early stage
- Typically produces symptoms of esophageal obstruction
- May appear as an irregularly narrowed and nodular, sometimes ulcerated, lesion simulating primary esophageal carcinoma
- Narrowing of the distal esophagus from spread of gastric cancer also may reflect malignant destruction of cells in the myenteric plexus (achalasia pattern)

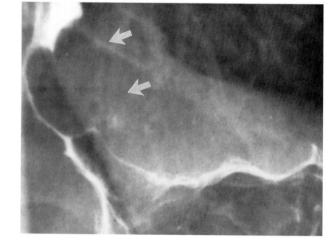

FIGURE 4-8

Direct extension of gastric cancer to involve the distal esophagus. Irregular tumor of the superior aspect of the fundus extends proximally as a large mass *(arrows)* that almost obstructs the distal esophagus.

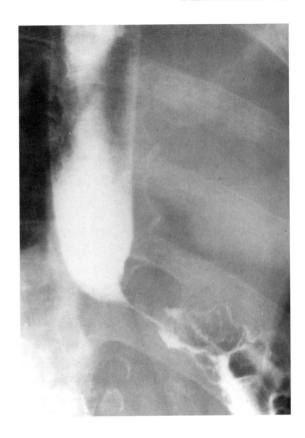

FIGURE 4-9
Achalasia pattern caused by the
proximal extension of gastric cancer.

Suggested Reading
Simeonne J, Burrell M, Toffler R. Esophageal aperistalsis secondary to metastatic invasion of
the myenteric plexus. *AJR* 1976;127:862.

Metastases to the Esophagus

KEY FACTS

- In the *cervical* region, direct extension from carcinoma of the larynx or thyroid
- In the *thoracic* region, carcinoma of the lung or breast may narrow the esophagus via tumor-containing lymph nodes or hematogenous metastases
- Symmetric stricture with smooth borders (occasionally irregular and ulcerated) that typically involves a short segment of the esophagus

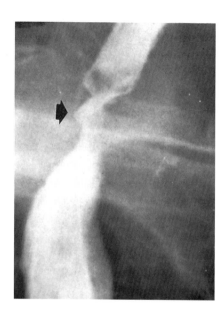

FIGURE 4-10

Metastatic thyroid carcinoma. Direct extension of tumor causes constriction and relative obstruction of the lower cervical esophagus *(arrow)*.

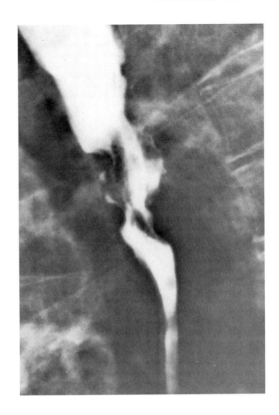

FIGURE 4-11
Metastatic gastric carcinoma. Irregular
ulcerated mass in the midesophagus.

Suggested Reading
Goldstein HM, Zornoza J, Hopens. Intrinsic diseases of the adult esophagus: benign and
malignant tumors. *Semin Roentgenol* 1981;16:183.

5 Other Disorders

Lower Esophageal (Schatzki) Ring

KEY FACTS

- Smooth concentric narrowing of the esophagus arising several centimeters above the diaphragm
- Usually asymptomatic, but may cause dysphagia if the width of the lumen is <13 mm
- Only visible if the esophagus above and below the ring is filled sufficiently to dilate to a width greater than that of the ring
- May represent a thin, annular peptic stricture secondary to reflux esophagitis

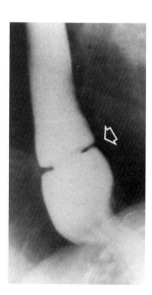

FIGURE 5-1

Lower esophageal (Schatzki) ring. Smooth concentric narrowing of the distal esophagus *(arrow)* marks the junction between the esophageal and gastric mucosae.

Suggested Reading

Schatzki R, Gary JE. The lower esophageal ring. *AJR* 1956;75:246.

Diverticula

ZENKER'S DIVERTICULUM

KEY FACTS

- Arises from the upper esophagus with its neck lying in the midline of the posterior wall at the pharyngoesophageal junction (about the C5-C6 level)
- Pulsion diverticulum that is apparently related to premature contraction or other motor incoordination of the cricopharyngeus muscle
- Small neck higher than the sac results in trapping of food and liquid within the diverticulum
- Large diverticulum may compress the esophagus and cause dysphagia or even esophageal obstruction

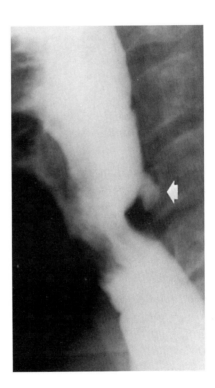

FIGURE 5-2
Zenker's diverticulum. Saccular outpouching *(arrow)* that arises just proximal to the posterior cricopharyngeus impression.

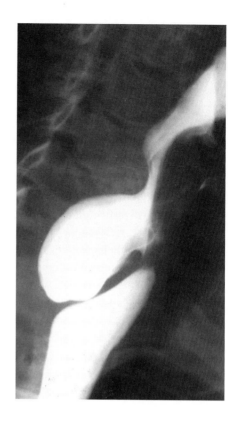

FIGURE 5-3

Zenker's diverticulum. Huge mass almost occludes the esophageal lumen.

Suggested Reading

Baron SH. Zenker's diverticulum as a cause for loss of drug availability: a "new" complication. *Am J Gastroenterol* 1982:77:152.

THORACIC DIVERTICULUM

KEY FACTS

- Arises in the middle third of the thoracic esophagus opposite the bifurcation of the trachea in the region of the hilum of the lung
- Traction diverticulum that develops in response to the pull of fibrous adhesions after mediastinal lymph node infection
- Often adjacent calcified mediastinal nodes from healed granulomatous disease

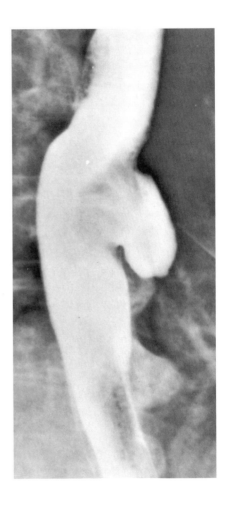

FIGURE 5-4

Traction diverticulum of the mid-thoracic esophagus.

Suggested Reading

Eisenberg RL. *Gastrointestinal radiology: a pattern approach.* Philadelphia: Lippincott–Raven Publishers, 1996.

EPIPHRENIC DIVERTICULUM

KEY FACTS

- Arises in the distal 10 cm of the esophagus and tends to have a broad, short neck
- Pulsion diverticulum that is probably related to incoordination of esophageal peristalsis and relaxation of the lower esophageal sphincter
- Small diverticulum may simulate an esophageal ulcer (though the mucosal pattern of the adjacent esophagus is normal)

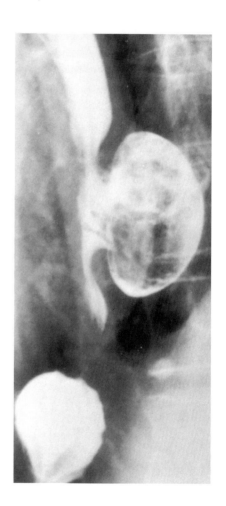

FIGURE 5-5
Epiphrenic diverticulum.

Suggested Reading

Bruggeman LL, Seaman WB. Epiphrenic diverticula: an analysis of 80 cases. *AJR* 1973;119: 266.

INTRAMURAL ESOPHAGEAL PSEUDODIVERTICULOSIS

KEY FACTS

- Multiple small (1–3 mm) ulcerlike projections arising from the esophageal wall

- The tiny necks may not fill completely, resulting in an apparent lack of communication with the esophageal lumen

- Involvement may be segmental or diffuse

- Pseudodiverticula represent dilated excretory ducts of submucosal esophageal glands, due to chronic inflammation (mimic Rokitansky-Aschoff sinuses of the gallbladder)

- Up to 90% have an associated smooth stricture in the upper esophagus

- Secondary infection with *Candida* is a common associated finding, but is not considered a causal factor

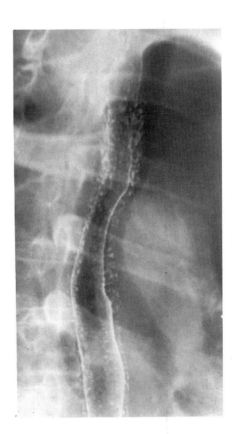

FIGURE 5-6

Intramural esophageal pseudodiverticulosis. Numerous diverticular outpouchings represent dilated ducts coming from submucosal glands in the wall of the esophagus.

Suggested Reading

Levine MS, Moolten DN, Herlinger H, et al. Esophageal intramural pseudodiverticulosis: a reevaluation. *AJR* 1986;147:1165.

Esophageal Varices

KEY FACTS

- Serpiginous filling defects (dilated venous structures) that change size and appearance with variations in intrathoracic pressure and collapse with esophageal peristalsis and distention
- "Uphill" varices in the distal esophagus are porto-systemic veins that enlarge because of portal hypertension
- Coronary vein collaterals connect with gastroesophageal varices that drain into the inferior vena cava via the azygous system
- "Downhill" varices in the upper esophagus result from obstruction of the superior vena cava (drainage from the azygos system through esophageal varices to the portal vein)
- On CT, enhancing vascular structures within and adjacent to the esophageal wall near the esophagogastric junction
- On MRI, vascular structures with signal voids due to flowing blood

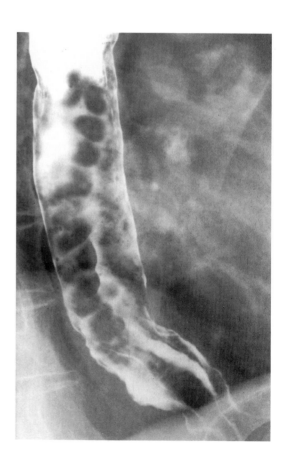

FIGURE 5-7

Esophageal varices. Serpiginous filling defects in a patient with portal hypertension.

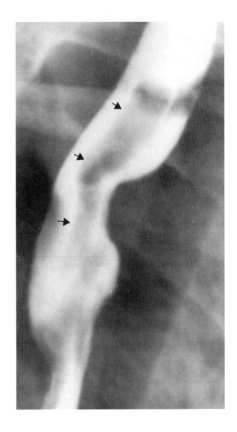

FIGURE 5-8
Downhill varices. Serpiginous filling defect
(arrows) in a patient with carcinomatous
obstruction of the superior vena cava.

Suggested Reading
Felson B, Lessure AP. "Downhill" varices of the esophagus. *Dis Chest* 1964;46:740.

Esophageal Foreign Bodies

KEY FACTS

- Usually impacted in the distal esophagus, just above the level of the diaphragm
- Other sites where foreign bodies tend to become impacted include (a) the cervical esophagus at or just above the level of the thoracic inlet, and (b) the level of the distal aortic arch
- Often a distal stricture, especially if the impaction is in the cervical portion of the esophagus
- Irregular margins may mimic an obstructing carcinoma
- Most metals are radiopaque and easily visualized on radiographs; objects made of aluminum and some light alloys may be more difficult to detect because their density is almost equal to that of soft tissue

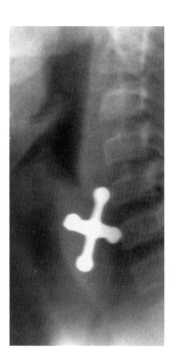

FIGURE 5-9
Metallic jack in the esophagus.

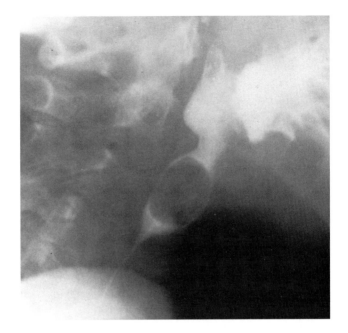

FIGURE 5-10
Cherry pit. The pit became
impacted in the cervical
esophagus proximal to a
caustic stricture

Suggested Reading

Webb WA. Management of foreign bodies of the upper gastrointestinal tract. *Gastroenterology* 1988;94:204.

Esophageal Perforation

KEY FACTS

- Major causes include:
  a. Emetogenic injury
  b. Closed chest trauma
  c. Iatrogenic (complication of endoscopy, stricture dilatation, bougie)
  d. Esophageal carcinoma
- In *Boerhaave's syndrome*, esophageal rupture is caused by severe vomiting that most frequently occurs in males and usually follows heavy drinking and a large meal
- *Traumatic* perforation of the thoracic esophagus leads to excruciating chest, back, or epigastric pain, accompanied by dysphagia and respiratory distress
- Chest radiographs demonstrate pneumomediastinum and subcutaneous emphysema of the neck, often with pleural effusion or hydropneumothorax
- Extravasation of contrast into the mediastinum and/or pleural space (virtually always on the left)
- Complications include acute mediastinitis, esophagorespiratory fistula, and superior vena caval obstruction

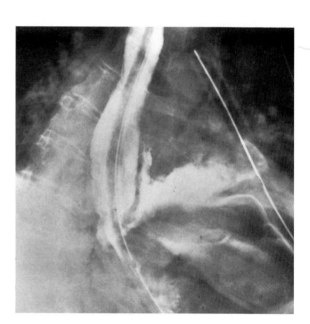

FIGURE 5-11
Boerhaave's syndrome. Note the extravasation of contrast material within the mediastinum and into the left pleural space.

Suggested Reading

Thompson NW, Ernst CB, Fry WJ. The spectrum of emetogenic injury to the esophagus and stomach. *Am J Surg* 1967;113:13.

Mallory-Weiss Syndrome

KEY FACTS

- Linear mucosal laceration at or near the gastric cardia due to a sudden, dramatic increase in intraesophageal pressure
- May cause massive hematemesis, though bleeding is usually self-limited and most tears heal spontaneously within 2 to 3 days
- Commonly missed on upper GI series (generally identified on endoscopy)
- May appear radiographically as a longitudinally oriented linear collection of barium in the distal esophagus, at or slightly above the esophagogastric junction

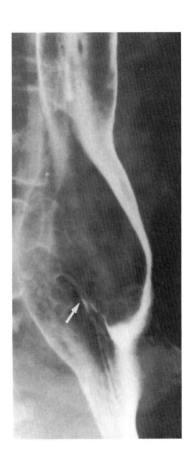

FIGURE 5-12
Mallory-Weiss tear. Linear collection of barium *(arrow)* in the distal esophagus, just above the gastroesophageal junction. (From Gore RM, Levine MS, Laufer I, eds. *Textbook of gastrointestinal radiology.* Philadelphia: WB Saunders, 1994, with permission.)

Suggested Reading
Carr JC. The Mallory-Weiss syndrome. *Clin Radiol* 1973;24:107.

Part B
DIAPHRAGM

6 Diaphragmatic Hernias

Hiatal Hernia

KEY FACTS

- Classic symptoms (heartburn, regurgitation, pain, dysphagia) reflect gastroesophageal reflux, though reflux often occurs in the absence of a radiographically detectable hernia
- Major complications include esophagitis, esophageal ulcer, and stenosis of the esophagus secondary to fibrotic healing of the inflammatory process
- Retention of food or refluxed gastric contents predisposes to pulmonary aspiration
- Plain chest radiographs may demonstrate a retrocardiac soft-tissue mass that often contains a prominent air-fluid level

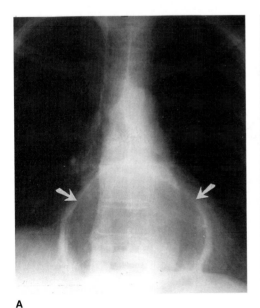
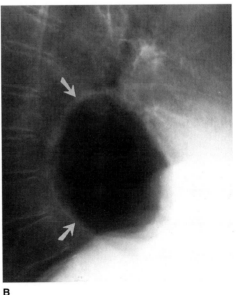

A

B

FIGURE 6-1   Hiatal hernia. Huge air-filled lesion appears as a mediastinal mass *(arrows)* on frontal (**A**) and lateral projections (**B**).

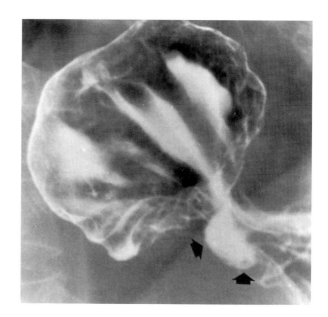

FIGURE 6-2
Hiatal hernia. Penetrating ulcer
(arrows) in a large hernia sac.

Suggested Reading

Govoni, Whalen JP, Kazam E. Hiatal hernia: a relook. *Radiographics* 1983;3:612.

Paraesophageal Hernia

KEY FACTS

- Progressive herniation of the stomach anterior to the esophagus (usually through a widened esophageal hiatus but occasionally through a separate adjacent gap in the diaphragm)
- Esophagogastric junction remains in its normal position below the diaphragm (unlike hiatal hernia) and thus no reflux esophagitis develops
- Often asymptomatic even when the entire stomach has herniated into the thorax
- Major complications are gastric volvulus and the development of a gastric ulcer at the point at which the herniated stomach crosses the crus of the diaphragm

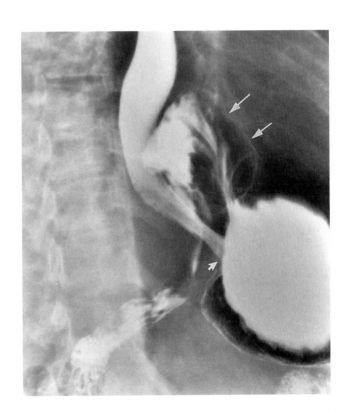

FIGURE 6-3
Paraesophageal hernia. Although a portion of the stomach *(long arrows)* is located within the hernia sac, the esophagogastric junction *(short arrow)* remains below the level of the left hemidiaphragm. Note the associated gastric volvulus.

Suggested Reading

Gerson DE, Lewicki AM. Intrathoracic stomach: when does it obstruct? *Radiology* 1976;119: 257.

Morgagni Hernia

KEY FACTS

- Herniation through the anteromedial foramen of Morgagni (usually on the right)
- Often associated with obesity, trauma, or other cause of increased intraabdominal pressure
- Typically appears as a large, smoothly marginated anterior mediastinal soft-tissue mass in the right cardiophrenic angle
- If the hernia contains only liver or omentum and no gas-filled bowel, it may be impossible on plain films to distinguish from a pericardial cyst or epicardial fat pad.
- Coronal MRI can demonstrate the diaphragmatic defect, thus excluding partial eventration of the hemidiaphragm

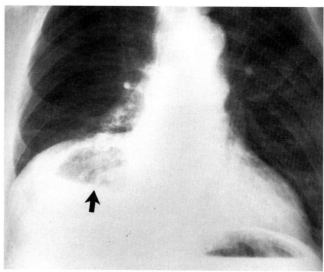

A

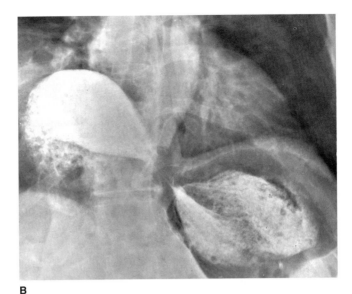

B

FIGURE 6-4

Morgagni hernia. **A:** Chest radiograph demonstrates a soft-tissue mass in the right cardiophrenic angle. In this projection, the gas within the mass *(arrow)* is in the inverted gastric antrum. The gas on the left is in the fundus. Frontal (**B**) and lateral (**C**) views with barium show typical herniation of the stomach through the right foramen of Morgagni with volvulus. The anterior position of the hernia is clearly visible on the lateral projection. (From Rennell CL. Foramen of Morgagni hernia with volvulus of the stomach. *AJR* 1973:117:248, with permission.)

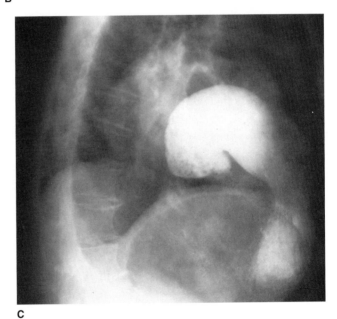

C

Suggested Reading

Rennell CL. Foramen of Morgagni hernia with volvulus of the stomach. *AJR* 1973;117:248.

Bochdalek Hernia

KEY FACTS

- Herniation through the posterolateral foramen of Bochdalek (usually on the left)
- Large hernias present in the neonatal period with hypoplasia of the ipsilateral lung and respiratory distress
- Typically appears as a large posterior mediastinal retrocardiac soft-tissue mass
- Generally contains opaque omentum, spleen, liver, or kidney, and may require contrast study or CT if there are no diagnostic air-filled bowel loops within the mass

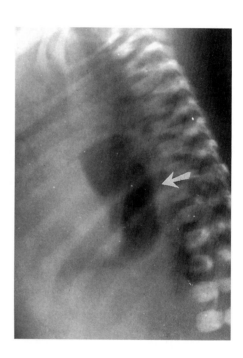

FIGURE 6-5

Bochdalek hernia. Gas-filled loop of bowel *(arrow)* is visible posteriorly in the thoracic cavity.

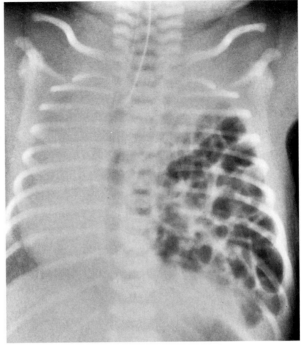

FIGURE 6-6
Congenital Bochdalek hernia. Frontal radiograph in a newborn infant with severe respiratory distress shows shift of the mediastinum to the right, caused by bowel herniated into the left hemithorax. At surgery, the hernia was repaired, but postoperatively the patient died because of severely hypoplastic lungs. (From Tarver RD, Godwin JD, Putnam CE. The diaphragm. *Radiol Clin North Am* 1984;22:615, with permission.)

Suggested Reading

Tarver RD, Godwin JD, Putnam CE. The diaphragm. *Radiol Clin North Am* 1984;22:615.

Traumatic Hernia

KEY FACTS

- Most commonly follows direct laceration, but also may develop as a result of any marked increase in intraabdominal pressure
- Should be suspected in any patient with a history of blunt abdominal trauma who develops vague upper abdominal symptoms
- Up to 95% of traumatic hernias occur on the left ("protective" effect of the liver on the right)
- Plain chest radiographs typically demonstrate herniated bowel contents above the expected level of the diaphragm (which often cannot be precisely delineated)
- Herniated viscera that appears to parallel the hemidiaphragm on both frontal and lateral projections can simulate diaphragmatic eventration or paralysis (contrast study may be required)

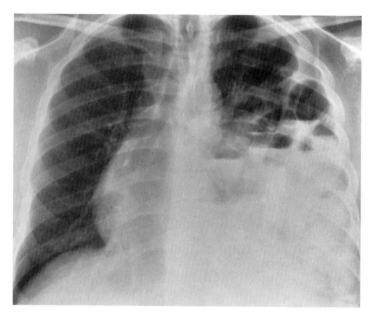

FIGURE 6 - 7   Post-traumatic diaphragmatic hernia. Plain frontal radiograph of the chest reveals herniated bowel contents above the expected level of the left hemidiaphragm.

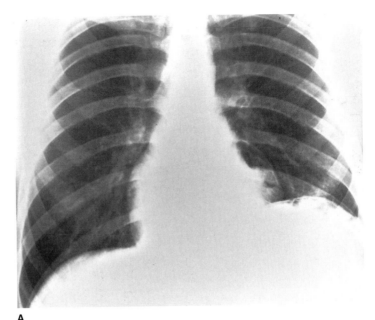

A

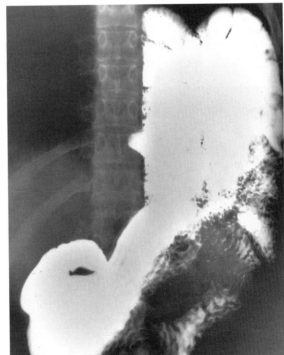

B

FIGURE 6-8
Post-traumatic diaphragmatic hernia. **A:** On the plain frontal chest radiograph, the elevation of the hemidiaphragm simulates eventration or paralysis. **B:** Administration of barium clearly demonstrates herniation of bowel contents into the chest.

Suggested Reading
Ball T, McCrory R, Smith JO, et al. Traumatic diaphragmatic hernia: errors in diagnosis. *AJR* 1982;138:633.

Part C
STOMACH

7 Peptic Ulcer Disease

Gastric Ulcer

BENIGN

KEY FACTS

- 95% of gastric ulcers are benign
- Related to *Helicobacter pylori* infection in 75% to 85% of cases
- Radiographic signs of benign gastric ulcer include:
  a. penetration (clear projection of the ulcer beyond the normal barium-filled gastric lumen on profile view)
  b. Hampton line, ulcer collar, or ulcer mound
  c. radiation of smooth thickened folds extending directly to the edge of the crater
  d. ring shadow (ulcer on the nondependent side on an en face view)
  e. halo defect (wide lucent band symmetrically surrounding the ulcer that resembles an extensive ulcer mound when viewed en face)
- Size, depth, and location of the ulcer (except for those in the cardia) are of no diagnostic value in differentiating benign from malignant gastric ulcers
- Most gastric ulcers heal completely with medical therapy (50% by 3 weeks; virtually all by 6 to 8 weeks)
- Only complete healing proves that a gastric ulcer was benign

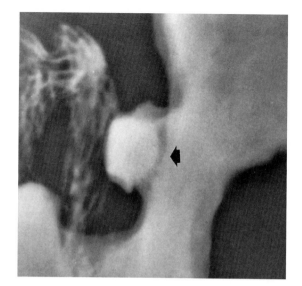

FIGURE 7-1

Benign gastric ulcer (penetration; ulcer collar). On this profile view, the ulcer crater penetrates well beyond the gastric lumen and is separated from the lumen by a lucent collar *(arrow)*.

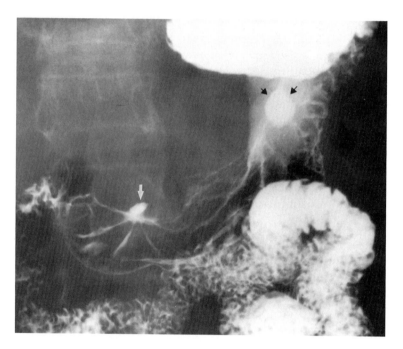

FIGURE 7-2   Multiple benign gastric ulcers (radiation of folds). The folds extend to the large ulcer, seen en face *(black arrows)*, and to the smaller ulcer, seen in profile *(white arrow)*.

Suggested Reading

Wolf BS. Observations on roentgen features of benign and malignant ulcers. *Semin Roentgenol* 1971;6:140.

MALIGNANT

KEY FACTS

- 5% of gastric ulcers are malignant
- Fundal ulcers above the level of the cardia are usually malignant
- Radiographic signs of malignant gastric ulcer include:
  a. ulcer located within the gastric lumen (does not project beyond the expected margin of the stomach on profile view)
  b. irregular, nodular tissue surrounding the ulcer (unlike the smooth edematous mound surrounding a benign ulcer)
  c. abrupt transition between the normal mucosa and the abnormal tissue surrounding a gastric ulcer
  d. irregular or nodular thickened folds that radiate to the tumor mass surrounding the ulcer
  e. Carman meniscus sign (semicircular or meniscoid ulcer with its inner margin convex toward the gastric lumen on profile view)
- Because partial healing may occur, any gastric ulcer that does not heal completely must be examined by endoscopy

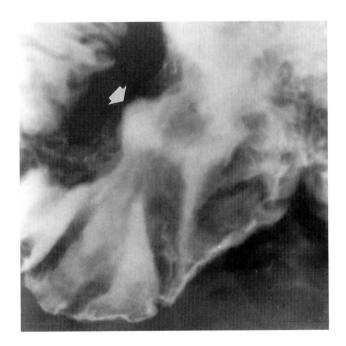

FIGURE 7-3
Malignant gastric ulcer. Thick folds radiate to an irregular mound of tissue around the ulcer *(arrow)*.

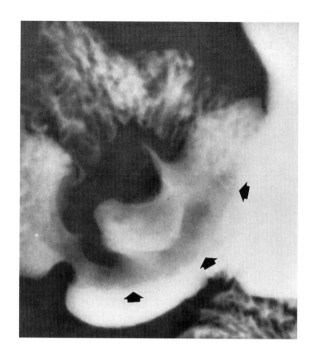

FIGURE 7-4

Malignant gastric ulcer (Carman meniscus sign). The huge ulcer has its inner margin convex toward the lumen and is surrounded by the radiolucent shadow of an elevated ridge of neoplastic tissue.

Suggested Reading

Carman RD. A new roentgen-ray sign of ulcerating gastric cancer. *JAMA* 1921;77:990.

Duodenal Ulcer

KEY FACTS

- Caused by excess duodenal acidity related to (a) abnormally high secretion of gastric acid and/or (b) inadequate neutralization
- More than 95% occur in the duodenal bulb
- Associated with *H. pylori* infection in >95% of cases
- Thickened folds, spasm, and deformity of the duodenal bulb are indications of peptic disease, but demonstration of the crater itself is necessary to diagnose an active duodenal ulcer
- Symmetric narrowing of the midportion of the bulb with dilatation of the inferior and superior recesses at the base of the bulb produce the classic cloverleaf deformity of a healed ulcer
- Once the diagnosis of duodenal ulcer disease is clearly established radiographically or by endoscopy, repeated attacks should be treated symptomatically, and there is no reason to repeat the upper gastrointestinal examination
- Complications of duodenal ulcer include obstruction, perforation, penetration (sealed perforation), and hemorrhage

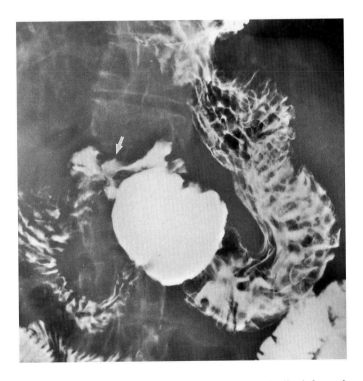

FIGURE 7-5   Duodenal ulcer. The large ulcer (arrow) lies within a markedly deformed bulb. Note the diffuse thickening of gastric folds in this patient with Zollinger-Ellison syndrome.

Suggested Reading

Peterson WL. *Helicobacter pylori* infection and peptic ulcer disease. *N Engl J Med* 1991;324:1043.

Giant Duodenal Ulcer

KEY FACTS

- Rigid-walled cavity that remains constant in size and shape throughout the gastrointestinal examination and lacks a normal mucosal pattern
- Most patients have moderate to severe abdominal pain, often radiating to the back, and a long history of prior ulcer disease
- May be overlooked by simulating a normal or deformed duodenal bulb
- High propensity for perforation and massive hemorrhage

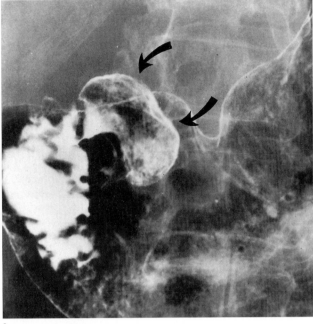

A

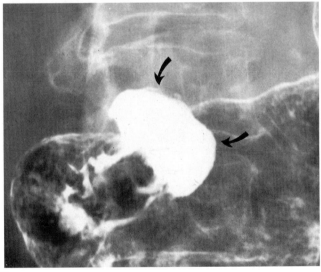

B

FIGURE 7-6   Giant duodenal ulcer. There is little change in the appearance of the
rigid-walled cavity *(arrows)* in air-contrast (**A**) and barium-filled (**B**)
views. (From Eisenberg RL, Margulis AR, Moss AA. Giant duodenal
ulcers. Gastrointest Radiol 1978;2:347, with permission.)

Suggested Reading

Eisenberg RL, Margulis AR, Moss AA. Giant duodenal ulcers. *Gastrointest Radiol* 1978;2:
347.

Postbulbar Ulcer

KEY FACTS

- Represents only about 5% of duodenal ulcers secondary to benign peptic disease
- Typically involves the medial wall just above the ampulla
- Although often difficult to detect radiographically, its identification is important because it frequently causes gastrointestinal bleeding, obstruction, pancreatitis, and atypical abdominal pain
- Severe spasm in the area of ulceration can narrow and deform the duodenal lumen and prevent barium from filling the ulcer crater

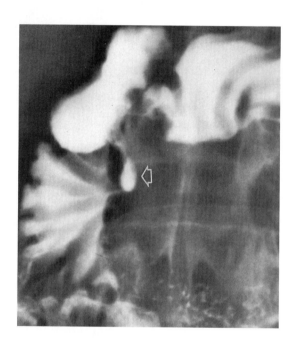

FIGURE 7-7

Postbulbar ulcer. Folds radiated to the margin of the ulcer *(arrow)*, which lies on the medial aspect of the second portion of the duodenum.

Suggested Reading

Kaufman SA, Levene G. Post-bulbar duodenal ulcer. *Radiology* 1957;69:848.

Zollinger-Ellison Syndrome

KEY FACTS

- Caused by a non-beta islet cell tumor of the pancreas (gastrinoma) that continually secretes gastrin (about 50% are malignant)
- Frequently a manifestation of multiple endocrine adenomatosis (especially involving the adrenals, parathyroids, and pituitary)
- Clinical syndrome includes (a) gastric hypersecretion and hyperacidity (elevated serum gastrin levels), (b) diarrhea or steatorrhea (due to inactivation of pancreatic enzymes by large volumes of acid), and (c) atypical recurrent peptic ulcer disease
- Suggested if duodenal ulcers are multiple or occur distal to the postbulbar region (though most ulcers in this syndrome occur in the duodenal bulb)
- Ulcers frequently fail to respond to traditional medical and surgical therapy for benign peptic ulcer disease
- Recurrent ulcers are characteristic after surgery and tend to occur at or distal to the anastomotic site (often lead to severe complications of hemorrhage or perforation)

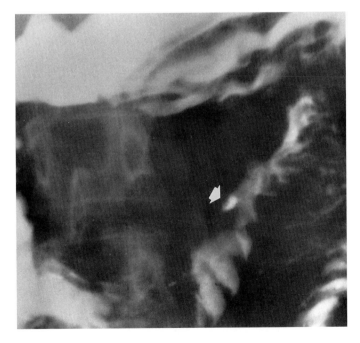

FIGURE 7-8   Zollinger-Ellison syndrome. Characteristic ulcer *(arrow)* in the fourth portion of the duodenum. Note the thickened gastric and duodenal folds.

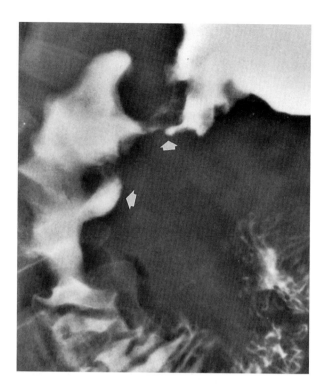

FIGURE 7-9
Zollinger-Ellison syndrome.
Bulbar and postbulbar ulceration
(arrows) in association with
diffuse thickening of folds in the
proximal duodenal sweep.

Suggested Reading

Zboralske FF, Amberg JR. Detection of the Zollinger-Ellison syndrome: the radiologist's responsibility. *AJR* 1968;104:529.

Complications of Ulcer Surgery

MARGINAL ULCERATION

KEY FACTS

- Postoperative complication of gastric surgery performed for the treatment of peptic ulcer disease
- Although they may develop within a few weeks of surgery, most marginal ulcers become symptomatic only within 2 to 4 years of partial gastrectomy
- Usually situated within the first few centimeters distal to the anastomosis
- Ulcers arising on the gastric side of the anastomosis are generally malignant
- Up to half of marginal ulcers are not detected radiographically (too superficial or shallow to be demonstrated or obscured by overlying barium-filled loops of bowel)

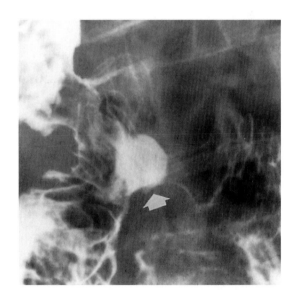

FIGURE 7-10

Marginal ulceration. This benign ulcer *(arrow)* is located at the distal portion of the Billroth-II anastomosis.

Suggested Reading

Jay BS, Burrell M. Iatrogenic problems following gastric surgery. *Gastrointest Radiol* 1977;2: 239.

BILE (ALKALINE) REFLUX GASTRITIS

KEY FACTS

- Thickened folds in the gastric remnant reflecting gastritis secondary to the reflux of highly alkaline bile and pancreatic juices into the stomach (normally prevented by an intact pylorus)
- Most severe changes tend to occur near the anastomosis
- May produce discrete reactive hyperplastic polyps (more likely than carcinoma if developing within a few years of surgery, though endoscopy and biopsy are required to confirm the diagnosis)
- Extensive swelling of gastric rugae can cause a mass effect

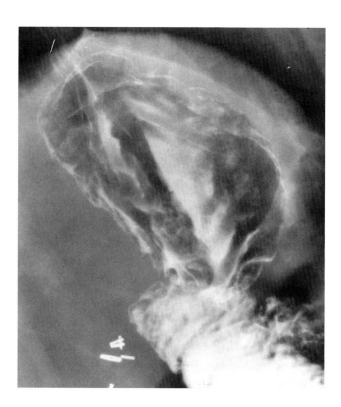

FIGURE 7-11
Bile (alkaline) reflux gastritis. Thickening of rugal folds in the gastric remnant following Billroth-II anastomosis.

Suggested Reading
Van Heerden JA, Priestly JT, Farrow GM, et al. Postoperative alkaline reflux gastritis: surgical complications. *Am J Surg* 1969;118:427.

GASTRIC STUMP CARCINOMA

KEY FACTS

- Malignancy occurring in the gastric remnant after resection for peptic ulcer or other benign disease
- Incidence of carcinoma arising in the gastric remnant following gastrojejunostomy is two to six times higher than in the intact stomach
- Develops at least 5 years after the original surgical procedure (more typically 10 to 20 years)

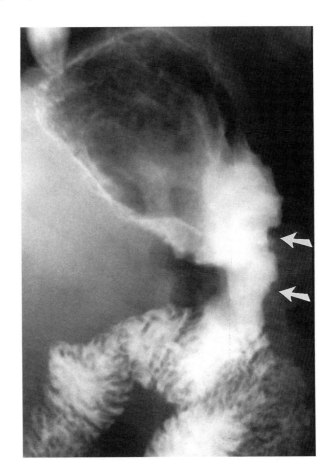

FIGURE 7-12
Gastric stump carcinoma. Irregular narrowing of the perianastomotic region *(arrows)*, which occurred 10 years after the original Billroth-II procedure for benign ulcer disease.

Suggested Reading

Burrell M, Touloukian JS, Curtis AM. Roentgen manifestations of carcinoma in the gastric remnant. *Gastrointest Radiol* 1980;5:331.

AFFERENT LOOP SYNDROME

KEY FACTS

- Partial intermittent obstruction of the afferent loop of a Billroth II gastrojejunostomy leading to overdistention of the loop by gastric juices
- Caused by mechanical factors (adhesions, kinking, intussusception), inflammatory disease, neoplastic infiltration, or idiopathic motor dysfunction
- Typically causes postprandial epigastric fullness relieved by bilious vomiting
- Upper GI series shows stasis of the proximal loop with preferential emptying of the gastric remnant into it
- CT shows rounded water-density masses forming a U-shaped loop in the region of the head and tail of the pancreas (oral contrast may fail to enter the loop)

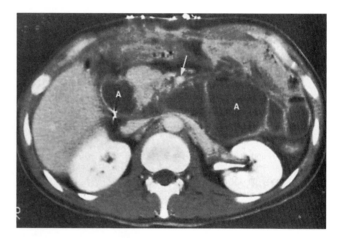

FIGURE 7-13   Afferent loop syndrome. CT demonstrates the abnormally dilated afferent loop *(A)* as multiple thin-rimmed cystic spaces seen adjacent to the pancreas and causing anterior displacement of the superior mesenteric artery *(arrow)*. (From Gore RM, Levine MS, Laufer I, eds. *Textbook of gastrointestinal radiology.* Philadelphia: WB Saunders, 1994, with permission.)

Suggested Reading

Swayne LC, Love MB. Computed tomography of chronic afferent loop obstruction: a case report and review. *Gastrointest Radiol* 1985;10:39.

8 Gastritis

Gastritis

HYPERTROPHIC

KEY FACTS

- Generalized thickening of folds that is most prominent in the fundus and body of the stomach
- Probably reflects a hypersecretory state and is often associated with peptic ulcer disease

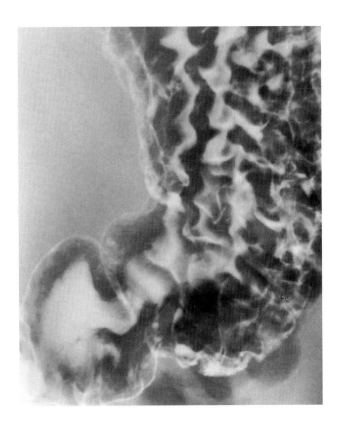

FIGURE 8-1
Hypertrophic gastritis. The patient had high acid output and peptic ulcer disease.

Suggested Reading
Press AJ. Practical significance of gastric rugal folds. *AJR* 1975;125:172.

ALCOHOLIC

KEY FACTS

- Generalized thickening of folds that usually subsides after withdrawal of alcohol
- Bizarre fold thickening may mimic malignant disease
- Relative absence of folds in chronic alcoholic gastritis

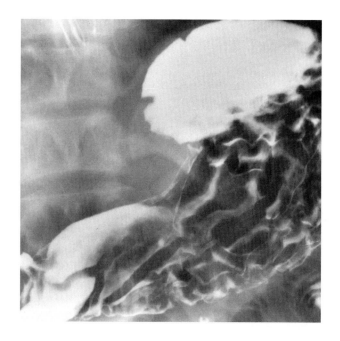

FIGURE 8-2
Alcoholic gastritis. Diffuse thickening of rugal folds.

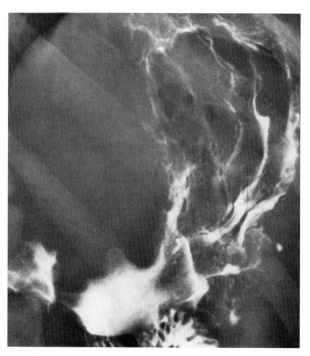

FIGURE 8-3
Alcoholic gastritis. Bizarre, large folds simulate a malignant process.

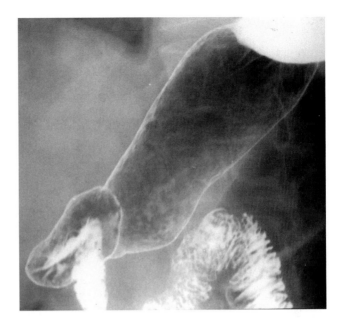

FIGURE 8-4
Chronic atrophic gastritis. Relative absence of folds in a patient with a long drinking history.

Suggested Reading
Levine MS, Palman CL, Rubesin SE, et al. Atrophic gastritis in pernicious anemia: diagnosis by double-contrast radiography. *Gastrointest Radiol* 1989;14:215.

CORROSIVE

KEY FACTS

- Predominantly distal involvement with associated ulcers, atony, and rigidity
- Ingested acids cause the most severe injury
- The pylorus is usually fixed and open (due to extensive damage to the muscular layer)
- Acute inflammatory reaction heals by fibrosis and scarring, which results in stricturing of the antrum within several weeks of the initial injury

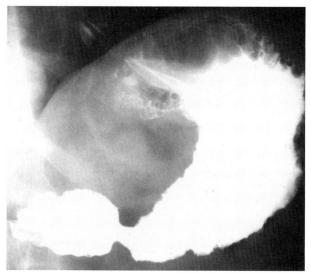

A

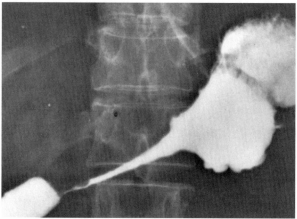

B

FIGURE 8-5   Corrosive gastritis. **A:** Diffuse ulceration involving the body and antrum due to the ingestion of hydrochloric acid. Note the widely dilated pylorus. **B:** Severe fibrotic stricture of the body and antrum, which developed within several weeks.

Suggested Reading
Muhletaler CA, Gerlock AJ, de Soto L, et al. Gastroduodenal lesions of ingested acids: radiographic findings. *AJR* 1980;135:1247.

INFECTIOUS

KEY FACTS

*   Due to bacterial invasion of the stomach wall or to bacterial toxins
*   Gas-forming organisms can produce gas in the stomach wall
*   Infection with the gram-negative rod *Helicobacter pylori* has been demonstrated in the stomachs of about 75% of patients with histologic evidence of gastritis (eradication of the organism by appropriate antibiotic therapy usually results in healing)

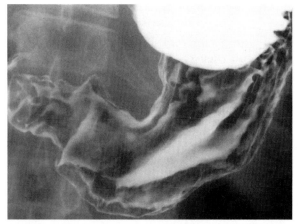

A

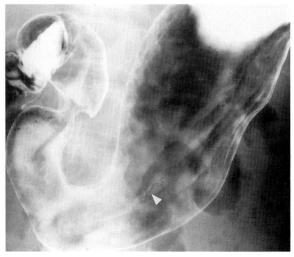

B

FIGURE 8-6   Anisakiasis. **A:** Diffuse fold thickening due to mucosal edema involves more the three-fourths of the gastric wall from the antrum to the body. **B:** The *arrowhead* points to the thin outline of the larva. (From Kusuhara P, Watanabe K, Fukuda M. Radiographic study of acute gastric anisakiasis. *Gastrointest Radiol* 1984;9:305, with permission.)

Suggested Reading

Dooley CP, Cohen H, Fitzgibbons PL, et al. Prevalence of *Helicobacter pylori* infection and histologic gastritis in asymptomatic patients. *N Engl J Med* 1989;321:1562.

Erosive Gastritis

KEY FACTS

- Superficial epithelial defects that do not extend beyond the muscularis mucosa
- A major cause is medications (aspirin, nonsteroidal anti-inflammatory drugs, steroids, alcohol)
- Crohn's disease and various infections (herpes, *Candida*, cytomegalovirus) can produce a similar appearance
- No etiology identified in half the cases (probably represent a manifestation of peptic disease)
- Small, very shallow flecks of barium surrounded by radiolucent haloes of edema
- The erosions tend to be aligned along the crest of nodularly thickened rugal folds (which may persist after the erosions have healed)

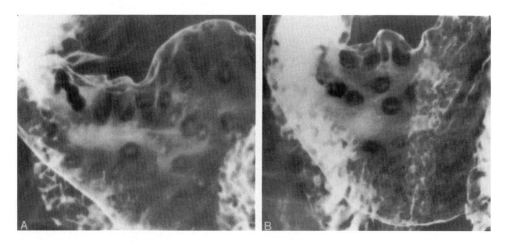

FIGURE 8-7   Erosive gastritis. Characteristic tiny barium collections, surrounded by haloes of edematous mucosa, in two different patients. (From Gore RM, Levine MS, Laufer I, eds. *Textbook of gastrointestinal radiology.* Philadelphia: WB Saunders, 1994, with permission.)

Suggested Reading
Poplack W, Paul RE, Goldsmith M, et al. Demonstration of erosive gastritis by the double contrast technique. *Radiology* 1975;117:519.

Crohn's Disease of the Stomach

KEY FACTS

- Almost always associated with concomitant ileocecal disease
- Typically involves the antrum (may progress to proximal portions of the stomach)
- Radiographic findings include:
    a. aphthous ulcers (punctate or slit-like collections of barium with a lucent halo, also seen in erosive gastritis)
    b. ram's horn sign (funnel-shaped antrum secondary to fibrosis)
    c. pseudo-Billroth-I sign (scarring of both the antrum and duodenal bulb with obliteration of the pylorus)

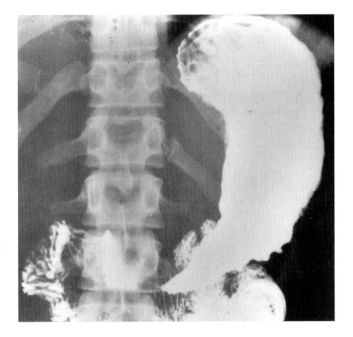

FIGURE 8-8   Crohn's disease. Smooth tubular narrowing of the antrum producing the "ram's horn" sign. (From Farman J, Faegenburg D, Dalemand S, et al. Crohn's disease of the stomach: the "ram's horn" sign. *AJR* 1975;123: 242, with permission.)

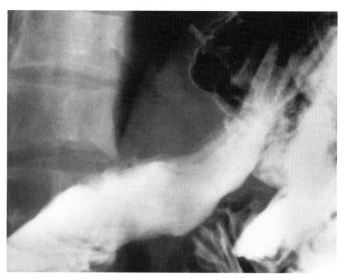

FIGURE 8-9   Crohn's disease. Pseudo-Billroth-I sign.

Suggested Reading
Farman J, Faegenburg D, Dalemand S, et al. Crohn's disease of the stomach: the "ram's horn" sign. *AJR* 1975;123:242.

9 Neoplasms

Gastric Carcinoma

KEY FACTS

- Third most common gastrointestinal malignancy (after colorectal and pancreatic carcinoma) and the sixth leading cause of cancer deaths
- Predisposing factors include (a) adenomatous and villous polyps, (b) chronic atrophic gastritis, (c) pernicious anemia, and (d) Billroth II gastrojejunostomy
- Radiographic appearances include:
  a. linitis plastica pattern (tumor invasion of the gastric wall stimulates a strong desmoplastic response that causes diffuse luminal narrowing)
  b. focal constricting lesion (simulating annular carcinoma of the colon)
  c. ulcerating mass
  d. polypoid mass (small malignant neoplasms may be indistinguishable from benign ones)
- CT is the imaging modality of choice for preoperative staging and treatment planning, as well as for assessing the response to therapy and detecting recurrence
- Metastatic spread:
  a. direct spread along peritoneal ligaments (to transverse colon, pancreas, liver)
  b. regional lymph nodes
  c. hematogenous (liver, adrenals, ovary, bone)
  d. peritoneal seeding
  e. left supraclavicular node (Virchow's node)

Suggested Reading
Levine MS, Kong V, Rubesin SE, et al. Scirrhous carcinoma of the stomach: radiologic and endoscopic diagnosis. *Radiology* 1990;175:151.

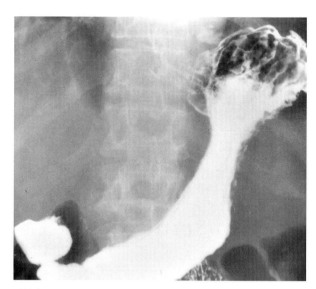

FIGURE 9-1
Carcinoma of the stomach.
Linitis plastica pattern.

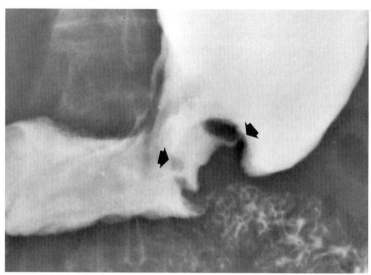

FIGURE 9-2 Carcinoma of the stomach. Huge ulcer in a fungating polypoid mass.

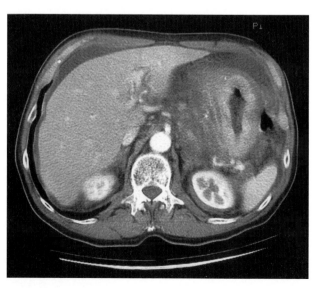

FIGURE 9-3
Carcinoma of the stomach. CT
scan shows marked thickening
of the gastric wall, which
shows contrast enhancement.
The extragastric extension and
ascites indicate tumor
dissemination with
intraperitoneal carcinomatosis.
(From Johnson CD, *Alimentary
tract imaging: a teaching file.*
St. Louis: Mosby-Year Book,
1993, with permission.)

Gastric Lymphoma

KEY FACTS

- 3% to 5% of gastric malignancies (primarily non-Hodgkin's lymphoma)
- Radiographic appearances include:
    a. large bulky polypoid mass that is usually irregular and ulcerated (often with substantial extragastric component)
    b. linitis plastica pattern (though unlike the rigidity and fixation of carcinoma, in lymphoma flexibility of the gastric wall is often preserved)
    c. diffuse or localized thickening of gastric folds (greater tendency to involve the distal stomach and lesser curvature than Ménétrier's disease)
- Associated splenomegaly and lymphadenopathy suggest the diagnosis
- High incidence of transpyloric extension into the duodenum (up to 33%); however, since gastric carcinoma (detectable involvement of the duodenum in about 5% of antral lesions) is 50 times more common than gastric lymphoma, transpyloric extension in an *individual patient* makes carcinoma the more likely diagnosis
- CT findings suggesting lymphoma rather than carcinoma include:
    a. more marked thickening of the gastric wall
    b. involvement of additional areas of the gastrointestinal tract
    c. absence of invasion of perigastric fat
    d. more widespread and bulkier adenopathy

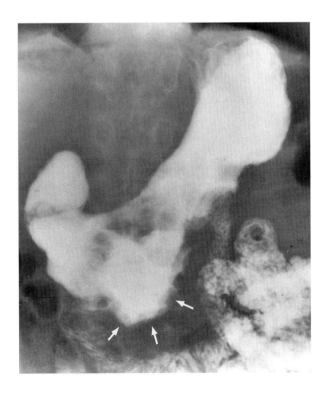

FIGURE 9-4
Lymphoma of the stomach.
Huge irregular ulcer *(arrows)* in
a neoplastic gastric mass.

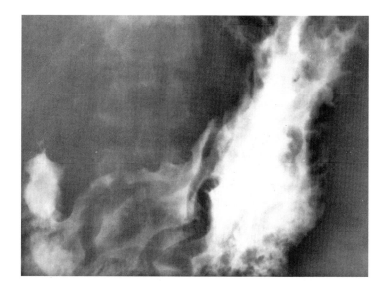

FIGURE 9-5   Lymphoma of the stomach. Bizarre irregular thickening of folds throughout the stomach.

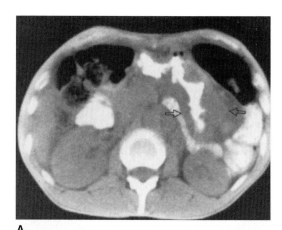

A

FIGURE 9-6

Lymphoma of the stomach. **A:** CT scan shows a circumferential intramural mass *(arrows)* causing gross distortion of the contrast-filled gastric lumen. **B:** The presence of large mesenteric *(N)* and periaortic nodes suggests the correct histologic diagnosis. (From Mauro MA, Koehler RE. Alimentary tract. In: Lee JKT, Sagel SS, Stanley RJ, eds. *Computed body tomography.* New York: Raven Press, 1983, with permission.)

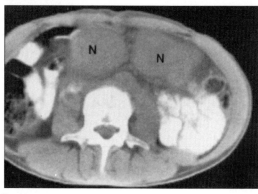

B

Suggested Reading

Marshak RH, Lindner AE, Maklansky D. Lymphoreticular disorders of the gastrointestinal tract. *Gastrointest Radiol* 1979;4:103.

Metastases to the Stomach

KEY FACTS

- Found at autopsy in <2% of patients who die of carcinoma
- May be hematogenous or lymphangitic spread, or by direct invasion (esophagus, colon, pancreas, kidney)
- Radiographic findings include:
  a. ulcerated "bull's-eye" lesions (melanoma, Kaposi's sarcoma, carcinomas of the breast or lung)
  b. submucosal nodules
  c. gastric wall thickening with circumferential narrowing of the lumen (direct extension from carcinoma of the pancreas or transverse colon, or desmoplastic hematogenous metastases from carcinoma of the breast)

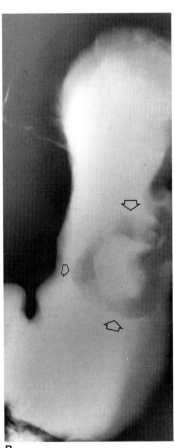

FIGURE 9-7

Metastases to the stomach. Ulcerated bull's-eye lesions from melanoma (**A**) and breast cancer (**B**).

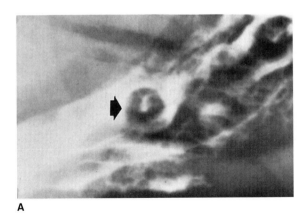

A

B

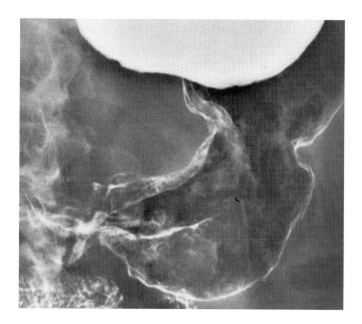

FIGURE 9-8   Metastases to the stomach. Hematogenous metastases from carcinoma of the breast produces scirrhous infiltration of the wall of the stomach, which causes narrowing of the lumen.

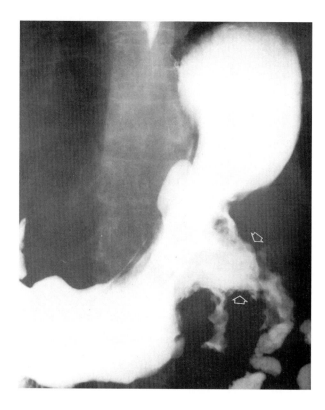

FIGURE 9-9

Metastases to the stomach. Direct extension from carcinoma of the pancreas produces a huge malignant ulcer *(arrows)* of the greater curvature.

Suggested Reading

Joffe N. Metastatic involvement of the stomach secondary to breast carcinoma. *AJR* 1975;123: 512.

Hyperplastic Polyps of Stomach

KEY FACTS

- Most common cause of discrete gastric filling defect (up to 90% of all gastric polyps)
- Small (1 cm), sharply defined, and often multiple
- Represents excessive regenerative hyperplasia in an area of chronic gastritis, rather than a true neoplasm
- Malignant transformation virtually never occurs (though there may be an independent coexisting carcinoma elsewhere in the stomach)

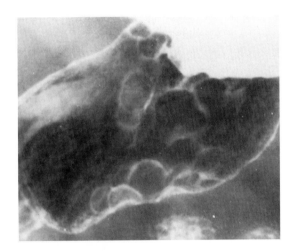

FIGURE 9-10

Hyperplastic polyps. Multiple smooth filling defects of similar size.

Suggested Reading

Feczko PJ, Halpert RD, Ackerman LV. Gastric polyps: radiological evaluation and clinical significance. *Radiology* 1985;155:581.

Adenomatous Polyp of Stomach

KEY FACTS

- About 10% to 20% of gastric polyps
- Large (≥1.5 cm), usually single, and sessile lesion with an irregular surface
- Active peristalsis may permit the development of a narrow long pedicle extending from the head of the polyp to the stomach wall
- Tends to develop in patients with chronic atrophic gastritis (as with hyperplastic polyps)
- One or more foci of carcinoma is found in about half of adenomatous polyps >2 cm (rarely in lesions <1 cm), all of which should be resected
- Increased incidence in patients with familial polyposis of the colon and the Canada-Cronkhite syndrome

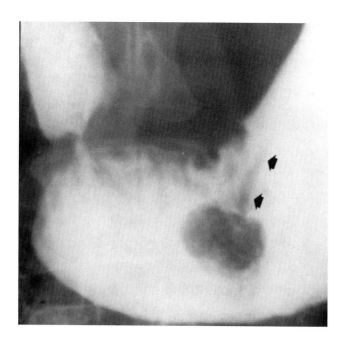

FIGURE 9-11

Adenomatous polyp. A long thin pedicle *(arrows)* extends from the head of the polyp to the stomach wall.

Suggested Reading

Op den Orth JO, Dekker W. Gastric adenomas. *Radiology* 1981;141:289.

Leiomyoma of the Stomach

KEY FACTS

- Most common benign spindle cell tumor of the stomach
- Typically produces a single intramural mass that often ulcerates (50%)
- Large lesions may have an extensive exogastric component suggesting malignancy
- Up to 5% demonstrate coarse calcification simulating uterine fibroids
- Multiplicity of tumors suggests malignancy, although evidence of metastases is often the only radiographic indication that the lesion is not benign

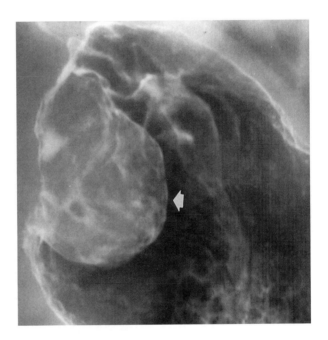

FIGURE 9-12
Leiomyoma. Smooth mass *(arrow)* in the fundus near the esophagogastric junction.

Suggested Reading
Kavlie H, White TT. Leiomyomas of the upper gastrointestinal tract. *Surgery* 1972;71:842.

Gastric Leiomyosarcoma

KEY FACTS

- Large bulky tumor typically found in the body of the stomach
- Although originally arising intramurally, leiomyosarcomas may present as intraluminal masses and often have a prominent exogastric component (suggesting an extrinsic lesion)
- Frequently undergo central necrosis, causing ulceration and gastrointestinal bleeding
- Often radiographically indistinguishable from benign leiomyoma (if there is no large exogastric mass)
- CT signs suggesting malignancy include:
  a. large size (>10 cm)
  b. central zones of low density (due to hemorrhage or necrosis)
  c. irregular pattern of enhancement

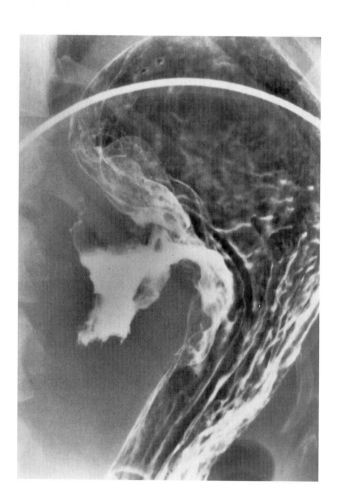

FIGURE 9-13

Leiomyosarcoma. Submucosal mass on the lesser curvature with a large and irregular ulceration. (From Nauert EC, Zornoza J, Ordonez N. Gastric leiomoyosarcomas. *AJR* 1982; 139:291, with permission.)

Suggested Reading

Nauert EC, Zornoza, Ordonez N. Gastric leiomyosarcoma. *AJR* 1982;139:291.

10   Pseudotumors

Gastric Pseudotumors

ECTOPIC PANCREAS

KEY FACTS

- Submucosal nodule of aberrant pancreatic tissue typically located on the greater curvature of the distal antrum close to the pylorus
- Central umbilication represents the orifice of an aberrant pancreatic duct rather than ulceration

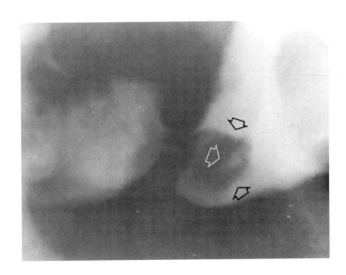

FIGURE 10-1
Ectopic pancreas. Filling defect in the distal antrum *(black open arrows)* with a central collection of barium *(white open arrow).*

Suggested Reading
Thoeni RF, Gedgaudas RK. Ectopic pancreas: usual and unusual features. *Gastrointest Radiol* 1980;5:37.

GASTRIC VARICES

K E Y   F A C T S

- Multiple smooth, lobulated filling defects in the fundus (tend to change size and shape during fluoroscopy)
- A single large fundal varix may mimic a leiomyoma
- Usually associated with esophageal varices and secondary to cirrhosis with portal hypertension (isolated gastric varices suggest splenic vein occlusion)
- On CT, well-defined clusters of round or tubular soft-tissue densities within the posterior and posteromedial wall of the proximal stomach

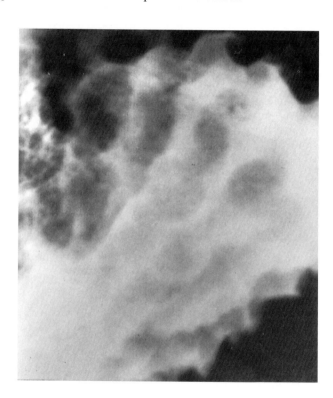

F I G U R E   1 0 - 2
Gastric varices. Multiple smooth, lobulated fundal filling defects represent the dilated venous structures.

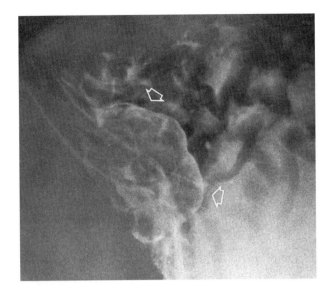

FIGURE 10-3

Gastric varix. Single fundal mass *(arrows)* in the region of the esophagogastric junction simulates a neoplastic process.

Suggested Reading

Balthazar EJ, Megibow A, Naidich D, et al. Computed tomographic recognition of gastric varices. *AJR* 1984;142:1121.

FUNDOPLICATION DEFORMITY (NISSEN REPAIR)

KEY FACTS

- Prominent filling defect at the esophagogastric junction that is generally smoothly marginated and symmetric on both sides of the distal esophagus
- Demonstration of a preserved esophageal lumen and mucosal pattern in addition to good delineation of the gastroesophageal junction should permit exclusion of a neoplastic process

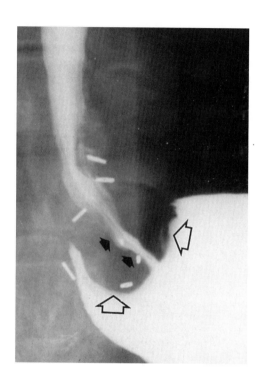

FIGURE 10-4

Fundoplication deformity (Nissen repair). The distal esophagus *(closed arrows)* passes through the fundal pseudotumor *(open arrows)*. (From Skucas J, Mangla JC, Adams JT, et al. An evaluation of the Nissen fundoplication. *Radiology* 1976;118:539, with permission.)

Suggested Reading

Skukas J, Mangla JC, Adams JT, et al. An evaluation of the Nissen fundoplication. *Radiology* 1976;118:539.

GASTRIC DIVERTICULUM

KEY FACTS

- Least common site of diverticula
- Diverticulum in the posterior portion of the fundus that fails to fill with barium or air may mimic a smooth-bordered submucosal mass
- On repeat examination, barium can usually be demonstrated to enter the diverticulum, thereby establishing the diagnosis

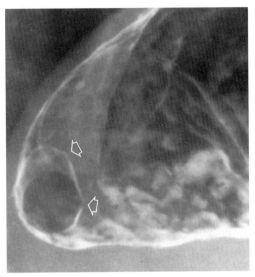

A

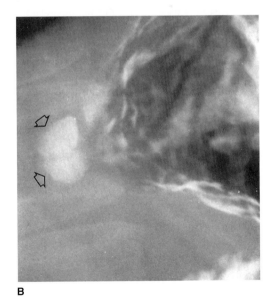

B

FIGURE 10-5
Gastric diverticulum. **A:** Gas-filled diverticulum *(arrows)* mimics a discrete fundal mass. **B:** On a later film, barium within the diverticulum *(arrows)* is clearly separated from the fundus, revealing the true nature of the process.

Suggested Reading
Freeny PC. Double-contrast gastrography of the fundus and cardia: normal landmarks and their pathologic change. *AJR* 1979;133:481.

DOUBLE PYLORUS

KEY FACTS

- Form of gastroduodenal fistula that consists of a short accessory channel connecting the lesser curvature of the prepyloric antrum to the superior aspect of the duodenal bulb
- Almost invariably associated with acute or chronic ulcer disease
- Formation of a second channel often results in reduction of ulcer pain (presumably due to improvement of gastric emptying)
- The two pyloric channels are separated by a bridge or septum of normal mucosa, which appears radiographically as a round lucency simulating a discrete filling defect

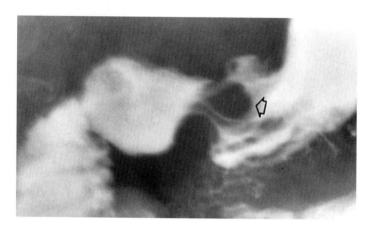

FIGURE 10-6   Double pylorus. The true pylorus and the accessory channel along the lesser curvature are separated by a bridge (septum), which produces the appearance of a discrete lucent filling defect *(arrow)*.

Suggested Reading

Einhorn RI, Grace ND, Banks PA. The clinical significance and natural history of the double pylorus. *Dig Dis Sci* 1984;29:213.

11 Other Diseases

Acute Gastric Dilatation

KEY FACTS

- Sudden and excessive distention of the stomach by fluid and gas, usually accompanied by vomiting, dehydration, and peripheral vascular collapse
- Within minutes or hours, a normal-appearing stomach can expand into a hyperemic, cyanotic, atonic sac that fills the abdomen
- Major causes include:
  a. abdominal surgery
  b. abdominal trauma
  c. severe pain or abdominal inflammation (renal or biliary colic, peritonitis, appendicitis, pancreatitis)
  d. immobilization (body cast, paraplegia)

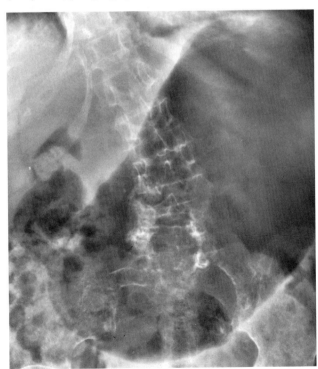

FIGURE 11-1
Acute gastric dilatation. Massively enlarged stomach that extends to the lower pelvis.

Suggested Reading
Joffe N. Some unusual roentgenologic findings associated with marked gastric dilatation. *AJR* 1973;119:291.

Bezoar

KEY FACTS

- Intragastric mass composed of accumulated ingested material
- *Phytobezoars* are made up of undigested vegetable material (classically associated with the eating of unripe persimmons)
- *Trichobezoars* (hairballs) occur almost exclusively in females, especially those with schizophrenia or other mental instability
- Bezoars developing in the gastric remnant are generally related to the eating of raw citrus fruits and can pass into and obstruct the small bowel (usually in the relatively narrow terminal ileum)
- Contrast material coating a bezoar and infiltrating the interstices may produce a characteristic mottled or streaked appearance

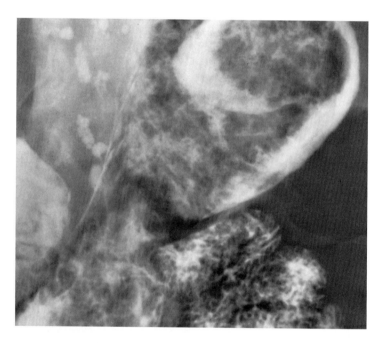

FIGURE 11-2   Bezoar. Infiltration of contrast into the interstices of the mass results in a characteristic mottled appearance.

Suggested Reading

Goldstein HM, Cohen LE, Hagne RO, et al. Gastric bezoars: a frequent complication in the postoperative ulcer patient. *Radiology* 1973;107:341.

Hypertrophic Pyloric Stenosis

KEY FACTS

- Idiopathic hypertrophy and hyperplasia of circular muscle fibers of the pylorus (with proximal extension into the gastric antrum)
- Classically produces bile-free projectile vomiting in a 6-week-old male
- Most common indication for surgery in infants
- Ultrasound findings include:
  a. target lesion (hypoechoic ring of hypertrophied muscle surrounding an echogenic center of mucosa and submucosa)
  b. muscle thickness >3.5 mm
  c. gastric outlet obstruction (lack of opening of the pyloric canal)
  d. elongated pyloric canal (≥17 mm)
  e. transverse diameter of the pylorus ≥15 mm

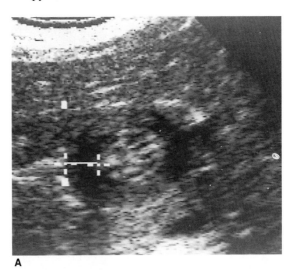

A

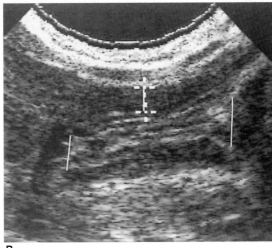

B

FIGURE 11-3
Hypertrophic pyloric stenosis.
A: Characteristic target lesion, consisting of a prominent anechoic rim of thickened muscle surrounding an echogenic center of mucosa and submucosa. The thickness of the muscle between the cursors measured 6 mm. **B:** On a longitudinal view, the elongated pyloric canal (between *vertical white lines*) measured 25 mm. Note the alternating echolucent and echogenic channels within the pyloric canal, corresponding to the "double track" mucosa sign on barium studies. The thickness of the pyloric muscle again measured 6 mm (between *cursors*).

Suggested Reading

Krebs CA, Giyanani VL, Eisenberg RL. *Ultrasound atlas of disease processes.* Norwalk, CT: Appleton & Lange, 1993.

Ménétrier's Disease

KEY FACTS

- Massive enlargement and tortuosity of rugal folds due to hyperplasia and hypertrophy of gastric glands
- Usually hyposecretion of acid, excessive secretion of gastric mucus, and protein loss into the gastric lumen
- Classically described as a lesion of the fundus and body, but may involve the entire stomach
- May be difficult to distinguish from lymphoma (lack of ulceration and rigidity, and the presence of excess mucus suggest Ménétrier's disease)

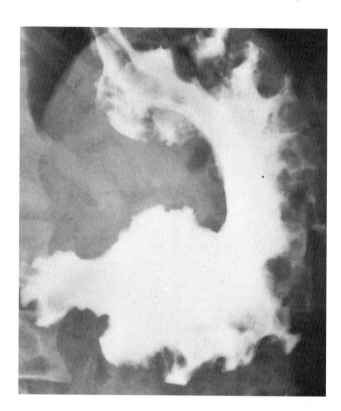

FIGURE 11-4
Ménétrier's disease. Generalized rugal fold thickening involves almost the entire stomach.

Suggested Reading

Olmsted WW, Cooper PH, Madewell JE. Involvement of the gastric antrum in Ménétrier's disease. *AJR* 1976;126:524.

Gastric Volvulus

KEY FACTS

- Uncommon acquired twist of the stomach on itself that can lead to gastric outlet obstruction
- Usually occurs in combination with a large esophageal or paraesophageal hernia that permits part or all of the stomach to assume an intrathoracic position
- *Organoaxial* volvulus refers to rotation of the stomach upward around its long axis so that the antrum moves from an inferior to a superior position
- *Mesenteroaxial* volvulus refers to rotation of the stomach from right to left or left to right about the long axis of the gastrohepatic omentum (line connecting the middle of the lesser curvature with the middle of the greater curvature)
- Radiographic appearances include:
  a. double air-fluid level on upright films
  b. inversion of the stomach (greater curvature above the level of the lesser curvature)
  c. positioning of the cardia and pylorus at the same level
  d. downward pointing of the pylorus and duodenum

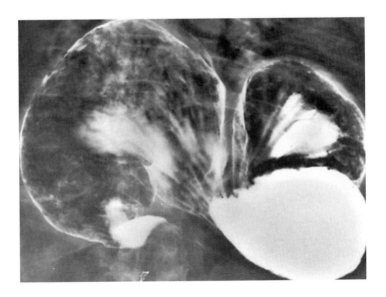

FIGURE 11-5 Gastric volvulus.

Suggested Reading

Gerson DE, Lewicki AM. Intrathoracic stomach. When does it obstruct? *Radiology* 1976;119: 257.

SMALL BOWEL

12   Malabsorption

Sprue

NONTROPICAL (IDIOPATHIC) SPRUE

KEY FACTS

- Classic disease of malabsorption characterized by diarrhea, steatorrhea, weight loss, anemia, and osteomalacia
- Diagnosis is made by jejunal biopsy, which demonstrates flattening, broadening, coalescence, and sometimes complete atrophy of intestinal villi
- Dramatic clinical and histologic improvement on a diet free of gluten (the water-insoluble protein fraction of cereal grains)
- Radiographic findings include:
    a. generalized dilatation of the small bowel (predominantly involving the jejunum)
    b. excessive amount of fluid in the bowel lumen (coarse, granular appearance of the barium, unlike the normal homogeneous quality)
    c. moulage sign (smooth contour and unindented margins of barium-filled loops of small bowel due to atrophy and effacement of mucosal folds)
    d. jejunization of ileal loops (long-standing disease)
    e. frequent episodes of transient intussusception

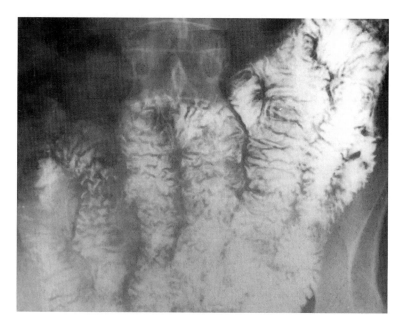

F I G U R E   1 2 - 1   Nontropical (idiopathic) sprue. Diffuse small bowel dilatation with hypersecretion.

Suggested Reading

Rubesin SE, Rubin RA, Herlinger H. Small bowel malabsorption: clinical and radiologic perspectives. *Radiology* 1992;184:297.

TROPICAL SPRUE

KEY FACTS

- Infectious process that responds well to folic acid and broad-spectrum antibiotics
- Radiographic and jejunal biopsy findings identical to those in nontropical sprue

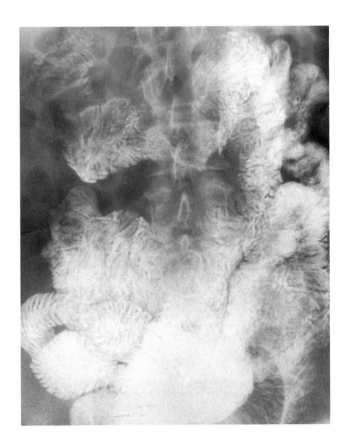

FIGURE 12-2

Tropical sprue. The barium in the dilated loops of small bowel has a coarse granular appearance due to hypersecretion.

Suggested Reading

Rubesin SE, Rubin RA, Herlinger H. Small bowel malabsorption: clinical and radiologic perspectives. *Radiology* 1992;184:297

Scleroderma

KEY FACTS

- Malabsorption related to prolonged intestinal transit time and bacterial overgrowth
- Characteristic skin changes, joint symptoms, and Raynaud's phenomenon usually precede changes in the small bowel
- Dilatation of the small bowel that is generally most marked in the duodenum proximal to the aorticomesenteric angle (entire small bowel may be diffusely involved)
- "Hidebound" pattern of thin folds that are sharply defined and abnormally packed together despite the bowel dilatation
- Pseudosacculations (large broad-necked outpouchings) may simulate small bowel diverticula

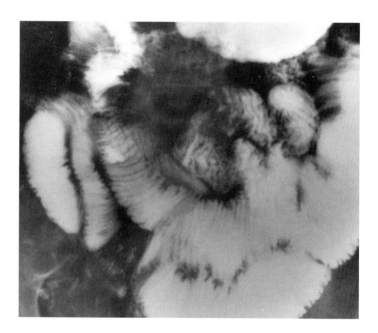

FIGURE 12-3   Scleroderma. For the degree of dilatation, the small bowel folds are packed strikingly close together (hidebound pattern).

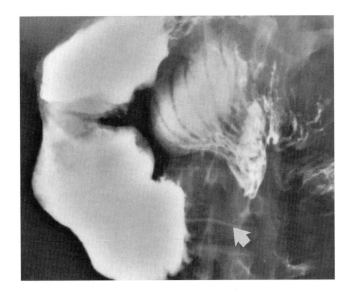

FIGURE 12-4   Scleroderma. Severe atony and dilatation of the duodenum proximal to the aorticomesenteric angle *(arrow).*

Suggested Reading

Horowitz AL, Meyers MA. The "hide-bound" small bowel of scleroderma: characteristic mucosal fold pattern. *AJR* 1973;119:332.

13 Inflammatory/Infectious Disorders

Ascariasis

KEY FACTS

- Roundworm that is the most common small bowel parasite
- After ingestion, complicated migration of larvae through the bowel wall, lung, and tracheobronchial tree to reach the alimentary tract again, where they mature into adult worms
- Complications include intestinal obstruction, peritonitis (if worms penetrate the bowel), biliary colic (if worms enter the bile duct), and hemoptysis (as worms pass through the lungs en route to the bowel)
- One or more elongated radiolucent filling defects (linear collection of barium may sometimes be seen filling the intestinal tract of the worm)
- A clump of coiled worms can produce a single intraluminal filling defect

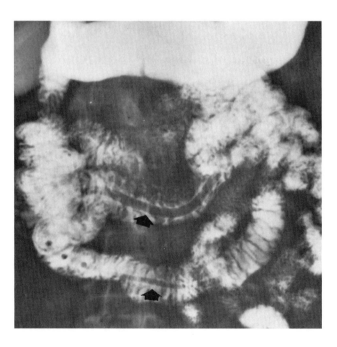

FIGURE 13-1

Ascariasis. The worms appear as elongated radiolucent filling defects *(arrows)*.

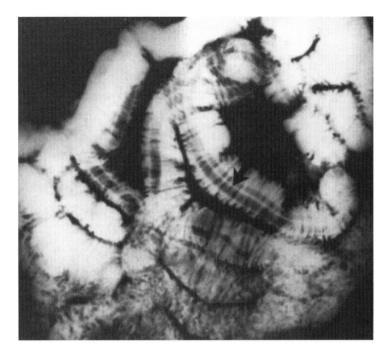

FIGURE 13-2   Ascariasis. The linear intestinal tract of the roundworm is filled with barium *(arrow)*. (From Gedgausas-McClees RK. *Handbook of gastrointestinal imaging.* New York: Churchill Livingstone, 1987, with permission.)

Suggested Reading

Weissberg DL, Berk RN. Ascariasis of the gastrointestinal tract. *Gastrointest Radiol* 1978;3: 415.

Crohn's Disease of the Small Bowel

KEY FACTS

- Diffuse transmural inflammation with edema and infiltration of lymphocytes and plasma cells in all layers of the bowel wall
- Broad spectrum of clinical appearances ranging from indolent course with unpredictable exacerbations and remissions to severe diarrhea and an acute abdomen
- Extraintestinal complications include large joint migratory polyarthritis, ankylosing spondylitis, sclerosing cholangitis, and renal oxalate stones
- Terminal ileum is almost always involved
- After surgical resection of an involved segment of bowel, high incidence of recurrent disease at the anastomotic site
- Radiographic findings include:
  a. generalized irregular thickening and distortion of small bowel folds
  b. cobblestone appearance (due to transverse and longitudinal ulcerations separating islands of thickened mucosa and submucosa)
  c. string sign (severely narrowed and rigid segment with loss of mucosal pattern)
  d. skip lesions (involved segments of varying lengths that are sharply separated from radiographically normal segments)
  e. separation of bowel loops (thickening of bowel wall and mesentery)
  f. mass effects on bowel loops produced by adjacent abscesses, thickened and indurated mesentery, or enlarged and matted lymph nodes
  g. fistula formation (to other parts of the gastrointestinal tract or other visceral organs)
- CT can also demonstrate thickening of the bowel wall, fibro-fatty proliferation of mesenteric fat, mesenteric abscesses, and lymphadenopathy

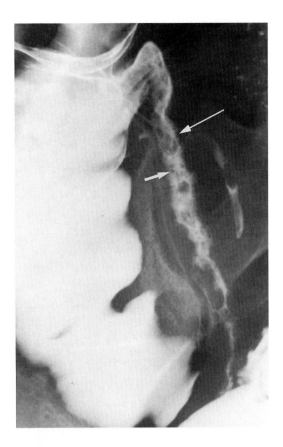

FIGURE 13-3

Crohn's disease. Compression view of the stenotic terminal ileum shows a diffuse granular mucosal pattern both en face *(arrow)* and tangentially *(arrowhead)*. (From Glick SN, Teplick FK. Crohn disease of the small intestine. Diffuse mucosal granularity. *Radiology* 1984;154:313, with permission.)

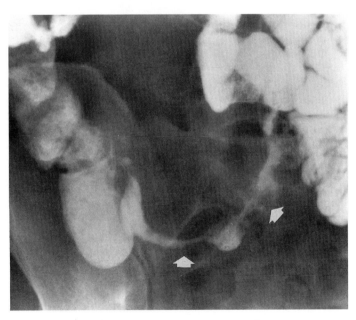

FIGURE 13-4 Crohn's disease (string sign). The mucosal pattern is lost in a severely narrowed, rigid segment of the terminal ileum *(arrows)*.

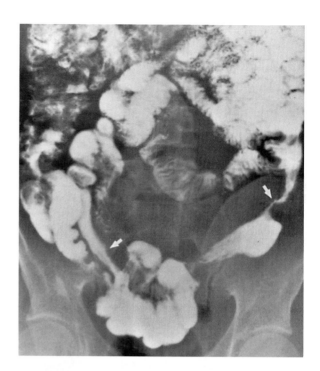

FIGURE 13-5
Crohn's disease (skip lesion).

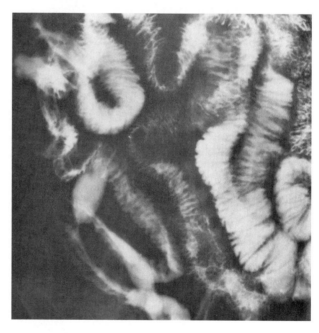

FIGURE 13-6
Crohn's disease. Separation of
small bowel loops is due to
diffuse mesenteric
involvement.

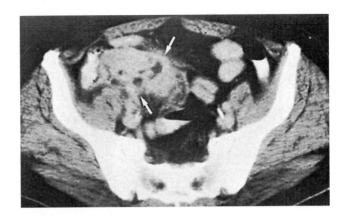

FIGURE 13-7
Crohn's disease. CT scan shows a large inflammatory mass *(arrows)* in the right lower quadrant. (From Gore RM, Levine MS, Laufer I, eds. *Textbook of gastrointestinal radiology.* Philadelphia: WB Saunders, 1994, with permission.)

Suggested Reading

Levine MS. Crohn's disease of the upper gastrointestinal tract. *Radiol Clin North Am* 1987;25: 79.

Eosinophilic Gastroenteritis

KEY FACTS

- Diffuse infiltration of the wall of the small bowel (and usually stomach) by eosinophilic leukocytes
- Irregular fold thickening that primarily involves the jejunum (though the entire small bowel may be affected)
- Peripheral eosinophilia and typical food allergies usually permit a precise diagnosis

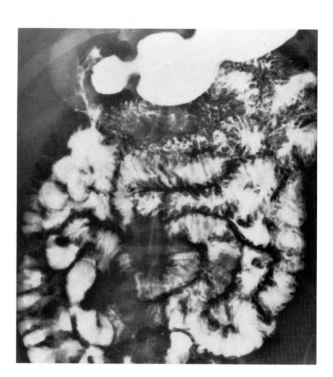

FIGURE 13-8
Eosinophilic enteritis. Irregular thickening of folds primarily involves the jejunum. No concomitant involvement of the stomach is identified.

Suggested Reading
MacCarty RL, Talley NJ. Barium studies in diffuse eosinophilic gastroenteritis. *Gastrointest Radiol* 1990;15:183.

Giardiasis

KEY FACTS

- Infestation by the protozoan parasite *Giardia lamblia* (harbored by millions of asymptomatic individuals throughout the world) from drinking contaminated water
- Clinically significant infections occur primarily in children, persons with altered immune mechanisms, and travelers to endemic areas (e.g., St. Petersburg, India, Rocky Mountains of Colorado)
- Irregularly thickened, distorted folds that are most striking in the duodenum and jejunum
- Hypersecretion, rapid transit time, and areas of spasm are often seen
- Small bowel pattern returns to normal after treatment with Atabrine (quinacrine) or Flagyl (metronidazole)

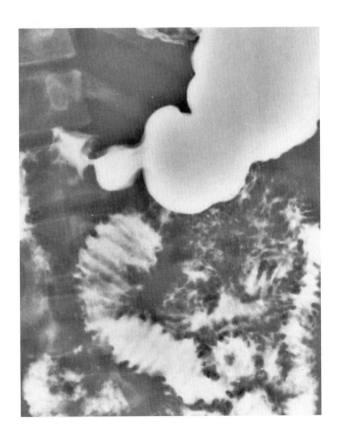

FIGURE 13-9
Giardiasis. Irregular fold thickening that is most prominent in the proximal small bowel.

Suggested Reading

Cevallos AM, Farthing MJG. Parasitic infections of the gastrointestinal tract. *Curr Opin Gastroenterol* 1993;9:96.

Strongyloidiasis

KEY FACTS

- Caused by the roundworm *Strongyloides stercoralis*, which lives in warm moist climates in areas where there is frequent fecal contamination of the soil
- Usually asymptomatic, but may cause severe abdominal pain, nausea and vomiting, diarrhea, weight loss and fever
- Irregular fold thickening primarily involves the duodenum and proximal jejunum (though severe infestation can involve the entire intestinal tract and be associated with toxic dilatation, spasm, ulceration, and stricture)

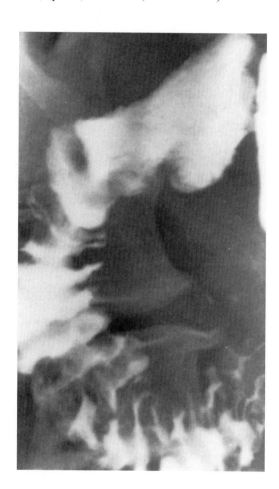

FIGURE 13-10
Strongyloidiasis. Irregular, at times nodular, thickening of folds throughout the duodenal sweep.

Suggested Reading

Dallemand S, Waxman M, Farman J. Radiological manifestations of *Strongyloides stercoralis*. *Gastrointest Radiol* 1983;8:45.

Tuberculosis of the Small Bowel

KEY FACTS

- May reflect (a) ingestion of tuberculous sputum, (b) hematogenous spread from a tuberculous focus in the lung, or (c) primary infection by cow's milk
- Fewer than half the patients have evidence of pulmonary tuberculosis
- Imaging appearance of small bowel involvement may be indistinguishable from that due to Crohn's disease (though tuberculosis tends to be more localized and predominantly affects the ileocecal region)
- Radiographic findings include:
  a. generalized, distorted, and irregular folds
  b. irregular narrowing of the bowel with separation of loops
- On CT, mesenteric adenopathy, peritoneal thickening, and high-density ascites

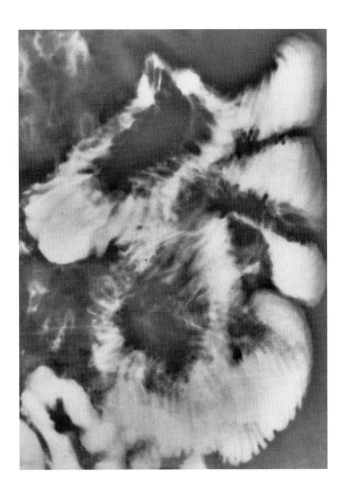

FIGURE 13-11

Tuberculosis. Separation of bowel loops, irregular narrowing, fold thickening, and angulation.

Suggested Reading

Carrera CF, Young S, Lewicki AM. Intestinal tuberculosis. *Gastrointest Radiol* 1976;1:147.

Typhoid Fever

KEY FACTS

- Acute, often severe, illness caused by *Salmonella typhosa*, which is transmitted by bacterial contamination of food and water by human feces
- Irregular thickening and nodularity of mucosal folds that is limited to the terminal ileum
- Mimics Crohn's disease, though in typhoid fever the ileal involvement is symmetric, skip areas and fistulas do not occur, and there is usually evidence of splenomegaly
- After treatment, the small bowel usually returns to normal (though healing with fibrosis and stricture can occur)

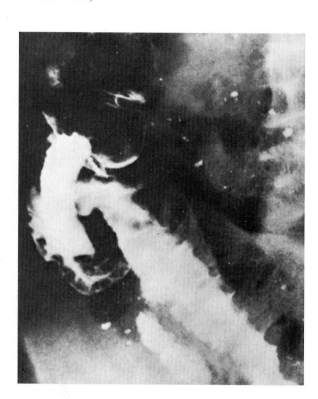

FIGURE 13-12
Typhoid fever. Thickened, coarse mucosal folds and marginal irregularity of the terminal ileum. (From Francis RS, Berk RN. Typhoid fever. *Radiology* 1974; 112:583, with permission.)

Suggested Reading
Francis RS, Berk RN. Typhoid fever. *Radiology* 1974;112:583.

Whipple's Disease

KEY FACTS

- Infiltration of the lamina propria by large macrophages containing multiple glycoprotein granules that react positively to the periodic acid-Schiff (PAS) stain
- Clinically, malabsorption syndrome and often extra-intestinal symptoms (arthritis, fever, lymphadenopathy)
- Irregular thickening of duodenal and jejunal folds with bizarre mucosal pattern
- On CT, characteristic low-attenuation lymph nodes in the root of the mesentery
- Small bowel appearance may revert to normal after antibiotic therapy

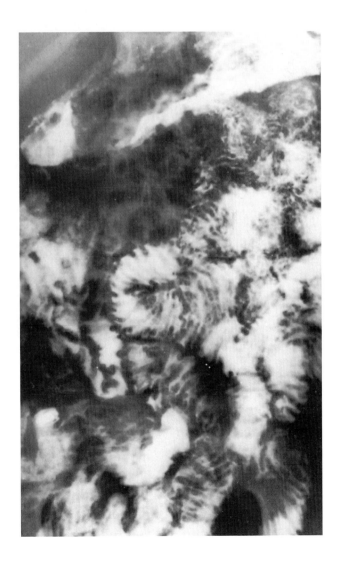

FIGURE 13-13

Whipple's disease. Diffuse irregular thickening of small bowel folds.

Suggested Reading

Philips RL, Carlson HC. The roentgenographic and clinical findings in Whipple's disease. *AJR* 1975;123:268.

Yersinia

KEY FACTS

- Gram-negative rod (*Yersinia enterocolitica*) that causes an acute enteritis with fever and diarrhea in children
- In adolescents and adults, acute terminal ileitis or mesenteric adenitis simulates appendicitis
- Predominantly a focal disease with coarse, irregularly thickened or nodular folds in the terminal ileum

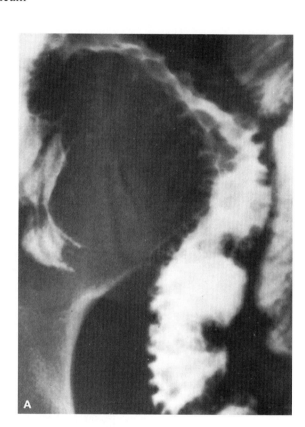

FIGURE 13-14

Yersinia. Numerous small nodules, marked edema, and moderate narrowing of the lumen combine to give the terminal ileum an appearance of irregularly thickened folds. (From Ekberg O, Sjostrom B, Brahme F. Radiological findings in Yersinia ileitis. *Radiology* 1977; 123:15, with permission.)

Suggested Reading

Gardiner R, Smith C. Infective enterocolitides. *Radiol Clin North Am* 1987;25:67.

14 Neoplasms

Lymphoma of Small Bowel

KEY FACTS

- May be primary or secondary (25% of patients with disseminated lymphoma have small bowel involvement at autopsy)
- Most frequent in the ileum, where the greatest amount of lymphoid tissue is present
- Radiographic findings include:
    a. infiltration of the bowel wall with thickening or obliteration of folds
    b. large, bulky polypoid mass with irregular ulcerations (may serve as the lead point for an intussusception)
    c. multiple large or small polypoid masses
    d. aneurysmal dilatation (secondary to tumor necrosis and muscle destruction)
    e. single or multiple extraluminal masses displacing adjacent bowel
- CT may show localized thickening of the bowel wall with exophytic and mesenteric tumor masses, in addition to lymphadenopathy and spread of tumor to the liver, spleen, kidneys, and adrenals

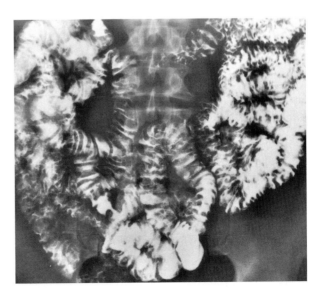

FIGURE 14-1

Lymphoma. Submucosal infiltration and mesenteric involvement produce a pattern of generalized irregular fold thickening and separation of bowel loops.

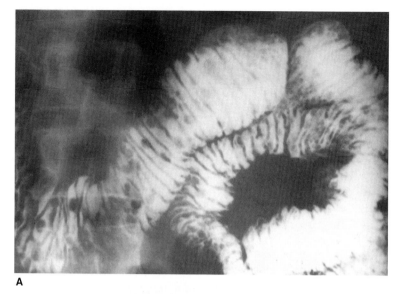

A

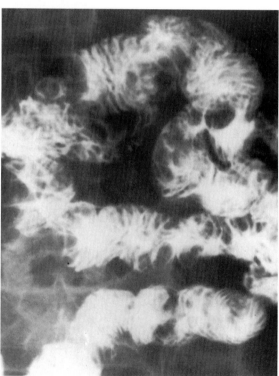

FIGURE 14-2

Lymphoma. Multiple small (**A**)
and large (**B**) nodular masses.

B

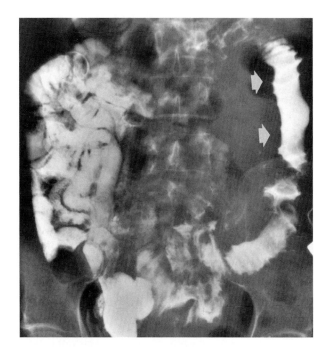

FIGURE 14-3
Aneurysmal lymphoma. Localized dilatation of a segment of small bowel *(arrows)* due to sloughing of the necrotic central core of the neoplastic mass.

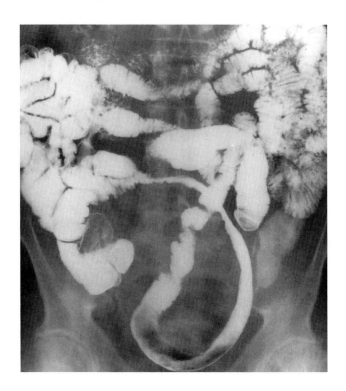

FIGURE 14-4
Lymphoma. Smooth narrowing of a segment of ileum, with obliteration of mucosal folds, displaced around a large suprapubic mass.

Suggested Reading
Zornoza J, Dodd GD. Lymphoma of the gastrointestinal tract. *Semin Roentgenol* 1980;15:272.

Carcinoid Tumor

KEY FACTS

- Most common primary neoplasm of the small bowel (especially involves the ileum)
- Low-grade malignancy that may recur locally or metastasize to lymph nodes, liver, or lung
- Rule of $1/3$ (frequency of metastases, second malignancy, and multiplicity)
- Presence of metastases is directly related to the size of the primary lesion (rare if <1 cm; about 90% if >2 cm)
- Carcinoid syndrome (due to serotonin) is found almost exclusively in those with liver metastases and consists of skin flushing, diarrhea, and abdominal cramps in addition to cyanosis, asthmatic attacks, and lesions of the tricuspid and pulmonic valves (about 7% of cases)
- Radiographic findings include:
  a. small, sharply defined filling defect (often missed radiographically)
  b. bizarre pattern of kinking, fixation, separation, and angulation of intestinal loops with diffuse luminal narrowing (due to intense desmoplastic response), with the small inciting tumor impossible to detect
- CT may demonstrate thickening, displacement, and kinking of bowel loops, a stellate radiating pattern of mesenteric neurovascular bundles, and enhancing liver metastases

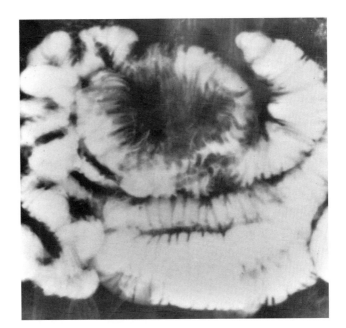

FIGURE 14-5

Carcinoid tumor. Separation of bowel loops, luminal narrowing, and fibrotic tethering of mucosal folds.

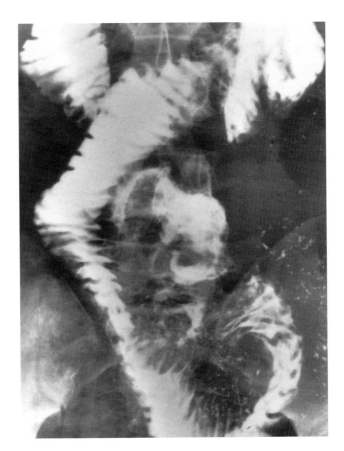

FIGURE 14-6

Carcinoid tumor. An intense desmoplastic response incited by the undetectable tumor causes kinking and angulation of the bowel and separation of small bowel loops.

Suggested Reading

Buck JL, Sobin LH. Carcinoids of the gastrointestinal tract. *Radiographics* 1990;10:1081.

Carcinoma of the Small Bowel

KEY FACTS

- Most common malignant tumor of the small intestine
- Primarily involves the duodenum and proximal jejunum (uncommon in the distal ileum, where most carcinoid tumors are found)
- Patients with sprue and Crohn's disease are at increased risk
- Tends to be aggressively invasive and extend rapidly around the circumference of the bowel, inciting a fibrotic reaction and luminal narrowing that soon cause obstruction
- Occasionally presents as a broad-based intraluminal mass; rarely appears as a pedunculated polyp

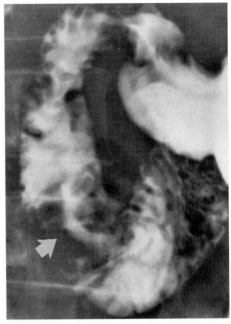

A

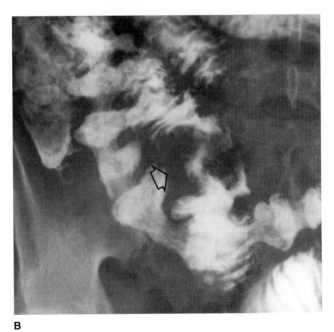

B

FIGURE 14-7
Carcinoma of the small
bowel. Annular constricting
lesions *(arrows)* of the
duodenum (**A**) and the ileum
(**B**).

Suggested Reading

Gore RM, Levine MS, Laufer I. *Textbook of gastrointestinal radiology.* Philadelphia: WB
    Saunders, 1994.

Metastases to the Small Bowel

KEY FACTS

- Most commonly hematogenous dissemination from melanoma, primary tumors of the breast or lung, or Kaposi's sarcoma
- May be direct extension from an adjacent neoplasm (ovary, uterus, colon, kidney, pancreas) or by intraperitoneal seeding (ovary, breast, gastrointestinal tract)
- Usually multiple filling defects, often with central ulceration (bull's-eye appearance)
- Other radiographic appearances include:
  a. large cavitating mass
  b. annular constricting lesion (may cause obstruction)
  c. separation of bowel loops with fixed and angulated segments
  d. extrinsic nodular impressions by mesenteric masses
- On CT, thickening of the bowel wall and mesentery

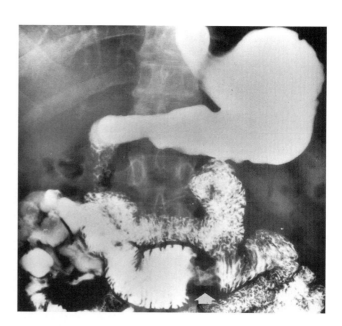

FIGURE 14-8
Metastasis to the small bowel. Annular constricting lesion *(arrow)* from a lung primary causes partial small bowel obstruction.

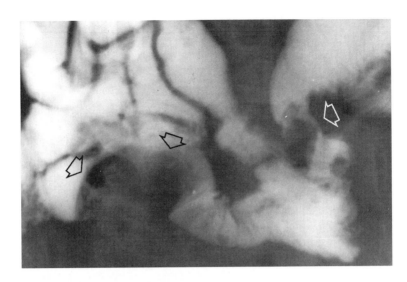

FIGURE 14-9   Metastases to the small bowel. Large mass impressions *(black arrows)* and an annular constricting lesion *(white arrow)* secondary to carcinoma of the breast.

Suggested Reading

Smith SJ, Carlson HC, Gisvold JJ. Secondary neoplasms of the small bowel. *Radiology* 1977;125:29.

Leiomyosarcoma of Small Bowel

KEY FACTS

- Large, bulky, irregular lesions that are usually >5 cm
- Tend to undergo central necrosis and ulceration, leading to massive gastrointestinal hemorrhage (and the radiographic appearance of an umbilicated lesion)
- Most tumors primarily project into the peritoneal cavity, so that their major manifestation is displacement of adjacent, uninvolved barium-filled loops of small bowel
- Spread by direct extension to adjacent structures and by the hematogenous route to liver, lungs, and bone (nodal metastases uncommon)

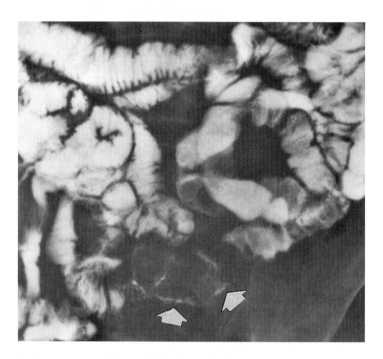

FIGURE 14-10   Leiomyosarcoma. Large, bulky, irregular lesion *(arrows)*.

Suggested Reading

Megibow AJ, Balthazar EJ, Hulnick DH, et al. CT evaluation of gastrointestinal leiomyomas and leiomyosarcomas. *AJR* 1985;144:727.

15   Other Disorders

Small Bowel Obstruction

KEY FACTS

- 80% of all intestinal tract obstructions
- Most common causes include postsurgical adhesions (75%), incarcerated external or internal hernias, malignancy, inflammatory disorders, intussusception, and gallstone ileus
- Radiographic findings include:
  a. markedly distended, gas-filled loops with a striking change in caliber when compared with bowel distal to the obstruction
  b. string-of-beads pattern of small gas bubbles in an oblique line (small amounts of gas in obstructed loops)
  c. sausage-shaped, dilated water-density shadows (if bowel proximal to an obstruction is filled with fluid and contains no gas)
- CT is the imaging modality of choice to diagnose small bowel obstruction and identify its cause

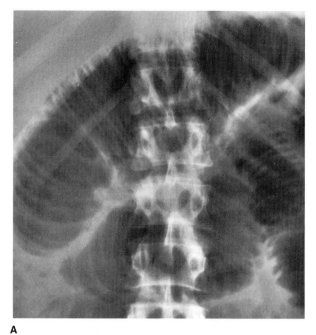

A

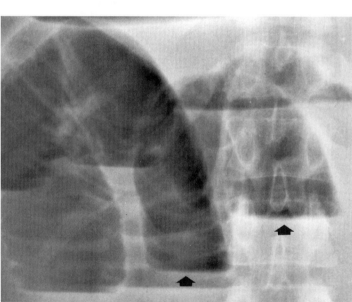

B

F I G U R E   1 5 - 1   Small bowel obstruction. **A:** Supine view shows greatly distended gas-filled loops of small bowel. **B:** On the upright view, the gas-fluid levels are at different heights within the same loop *(arrowheads)*.

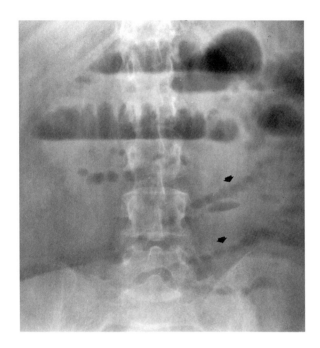

FIGURE 15-2

Small bowel obstruction. String-of-beads appearance *(arrows)*.

Suggested Reading

Frager D, Medwid SW, Baer JW, et al. CT of small bowel obstruction: value in establishing the diagnosis and determining the degree and cause. *AJR* 1994;162:37.

STRANGULATED OBSTRUCTION

KEY FACTS

- Complete or partial small bowel obstruction with impairment of the blood supply
- In closed-loop obstruction, both the afferent and efferent limbs of a bowel loop become obstructed
- Often difficult to diagnose radiographically, but if untreated can rapidly lead to hemorrhagic infarction and gangrenous bowel and perforation into the peritoneal cavity
- CT findings of *strangulation* include:
  a. circumferential thickening and high attenuation of the intestinal wall (consistent with ischemic or infarcted bowel)
  b. target sign (three concentric rings of high and low attenuation of the bowel wall affecting one intestinal segment)
- CT findings of *closed loop obstruction* include:
  a. fluid-filled distended loops that have a U-shaped configuration on longitudinal sections and a corresponding radial distribution on cross section
  b. stretching and thickening of mesenteric vessels, which converge toward the point of obstruction where they produce fusiform tapering (beak sign)

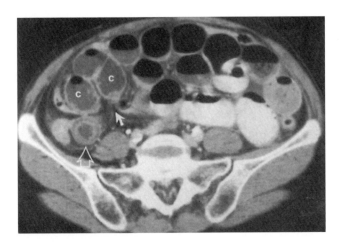

FIGURE 15-3   Strangulated obstruction (adhesions and volvulus). CT scan shows the fluid-filled closed loop *(c)* and three concentric rings of high and low attenuation of the bowel wall (target sign) that affect one intestinal segment *(open arrow)*. Note the discrepancy between the distended but mainly gas-filled proximal intestine and the fluid-filled closed loop *(c)*. The afferent and efferent limbs of bowel leading into the site of torsion *(solid arrow)* are tapered and adjacent to each other (beak sign). (From Balthazar EJ, Birnbaum BA, Megibow AJ, et al. Closed-loop and strangulating intestinal obstruction: CT signs. *Radiology* 1992;185:769, with permission.)

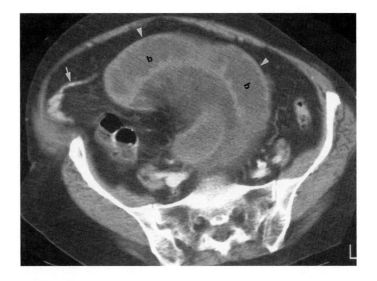

FIGURE 15-4   Strangulated obstruction (volvulus). Distended fluid-filled distal loop
of small bowel *(b)*, with a slightly thickened wall *(arrowheads)* and a
U-shaped configuration. The distal ileum *(arrow)* is completely
collapsed, a finding consistent with mechanical intestinal obstruction.
The attached mesentery has increased attenuation, with complete
obliteration of the mesenteric vascular markings. (From Balthazar EJ,
Birnbaum BA, Megibow AJ, et al. Closed-loop and strangulating
intestinal obstruction: CT signs. *Radiology* 1992;185:769, with
permission.)

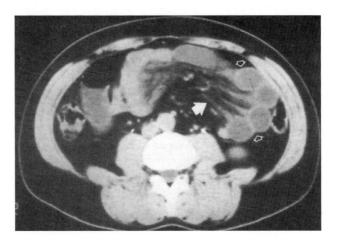

FIGURE 15-5   Strangulated obstruction (volvulus). Radial distribution of several
distended and fluid-filled bowel loops *(open arrows)*. Note the slightly
engorged and stretched mesenteric vascular structures *(solid arrow)*
converging toward the point of torsion. (From Balthazar EJ, Birnbaum
BA, Megibow AJ, et al. Closed-loop and strangulating intestinal
obstruction: CT signs. *Radiology* 1992;185:769, with permission.)

Suggested Reading

Balthazar EJ, Birnbaum BA, Megibow AJ, et al. Closed-loop and strangulating intestinal
obstruction: CT signs. *Radiology* 1992;185:769.

Gallstone Ileus

KEY FACTS

- Classic triad of:
  a. jejunal or ileal filling defect
  b. gas or barium in the biliary tree
  c. small bowel obstruction
- Caused by a large gallstone that enters the small bowel via a fistula from the gallbladder or common bile duct to the duodenum
- Usually occurs in elderly women

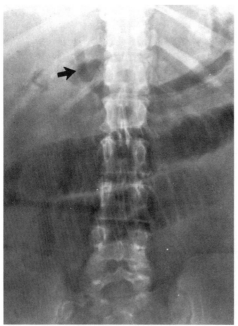

A

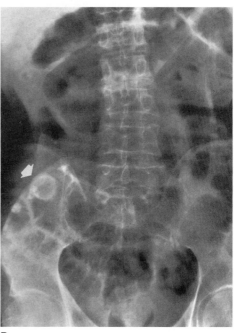

B

FIGURE 15-6   Gallstone ileus. Dilated gas-filled loops of small bowel that are combined with gas in the biliary tree *(arrow)* **(A)** and extend to the level of an obstructing gallstone in the ileum *(arrow)* **(B).**

Suggested Reading

Eisenman JI, Finck EJ, O'Loughlin BJ. Gallstone ileus. *AJR* 1967;101:361.

Adynamic Ileus

KEY FACTS

- Failure of fluid and gas to progress through a nonobstructed bowel because of decreased or absent peristalsis
- Major causes include:
  - a. drugs (atropine, glucagon, morphine, barbiturates, phenothiazines)
  - b. trauma, surgery
  - c. inflammation (peritonitis, pancreatitis, appendicitis, cholecystitis, abscess)
  - d. metabolic (diabetes, hypokalemia, hypothyroidism, hypercalcemia)
- Diffuse, uniform, predominantly gaseous distention of the entire small and large bowel without a demonstrable point of obstruction
- Occasionally, a gasless abdomen with dilated loops of bowel that are filled only with fluid

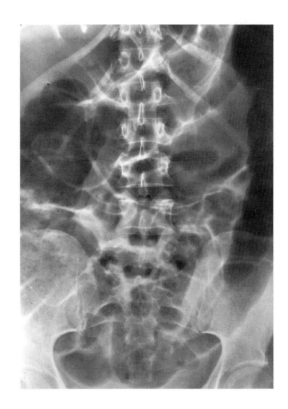

FIGURE 15-7
Adynamic ileus. Large amounts of gas within dilated loops of both small and large bowel with no demonstrable point of obstruction.

Suggested Reading
Livingston EH, Passaro EP. Postoperative ileus. *Dig Dis Sci* 1990;35:121.

FOCAL ILEUS (SENTINEL LOOP)

KEY FACTS

- Isolated segment of bowel that becomes paralyzed and distended because it lies adjacent to an acute inflammatory process
- The position of the sentinel loop suggests the underlying diagnosis:
    a. right upper quadrant—acute cholecystitis, hepatitis, pyelonephritis
    b. right lower quadrant—acute appendicitis, Crohn's disease
    c. left upper quadrant—pancreatitis, pyelonephritis, splenic injury
    d. left lower quadrant—diverticulitis
    e. midabdomen—pancreatitis

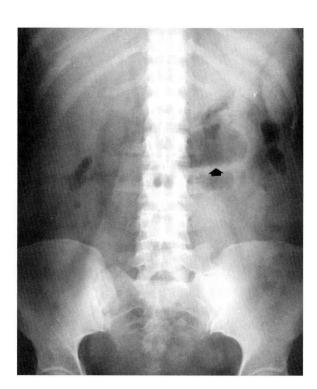

FIGURE 15-8
Focal ileus. Sentinel loop *(arrow)* in the mid-abdomen in a patient with acute pancreatitis.

COLONIC ILEUS

KEY FACTS

- Selective or disproportionate gaseous distention of the large bowel without any organic obstruction
- Massive distention of the cecum (often horizontally oriented) characteristically dominates the radiographic appearance
- Usually accompanies or follows an acute abdominal inflammatory process or abdominal surgery (but can occur with any of the causes of adynamic ileus)

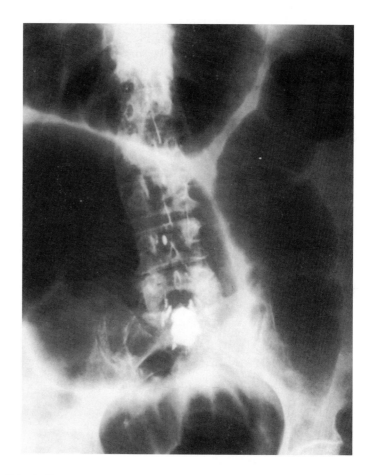

FIGURE 15-9   Colonic ileus. Pronounced dilatation of the colon in a patient with severe diabetes and hypokalemia.

Suggested Reading

Meyers MA. Colonic ileus. *Gastrointest Radiol* 1977;2:37.

Duodenal Atresia

KEY FACTS

- Complete obliteration of the lumen (most common cause of congenital duodenal obstruction)
- Second most common site of gastrointestinal atresia (after the ileum)
- Frequent vomiting and consequent loss of fluid and electrolytes can cause rapid clinical deterioration unless a surgical diverting procedure is performed promptly
- Relatively high incidence in infants with Down syndrome
- Radiographic findings include:
    a. Double-bubble sign
    b. Absence of gas in the small and large bowel (distal to the point of obstruction)
- Fetal ultrasound findings include:
    a. Polyhydramnios
    b. Double-bubble sign—simultaneous distention of the stomach and proximal duodenum with demonstration of continuity between them (usually not identified prior to 24 weeks gestational age)

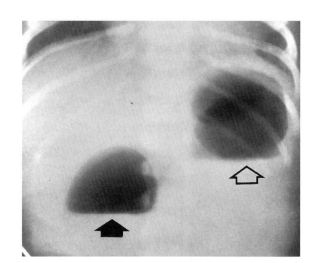

FIGURE 15-10
Duodenal atresia (double-bubble sign). The left bubble *(open arrow)* represents air in the stomach; the right bubble *(solid arrow)* reflects duodenal gas. There is no gas in the small or large bowel distal to the level of the complete obstruction.

Suggested Reading

Fonkalsrud EW, DeLorimier AA, Hays DM. Congenital atresia and stenosis of the duodenum. *Pediatrics* 1969;43:79.

Annular Pancreas

KEY FACTS

- Anomalous ring of pancreatic tissue encircling the duodenal lumen, usually at or above the level of the ampulla of Vater
- Incomplete obstruction (unlike complete obstruction in duodenal atresia)
- Relatively high incidence in infants with Down syndrome
- Radiographic findings include:
  a. double-bubble sign
  b. small but recognizable amount of gas distal to the high-grade stenosis

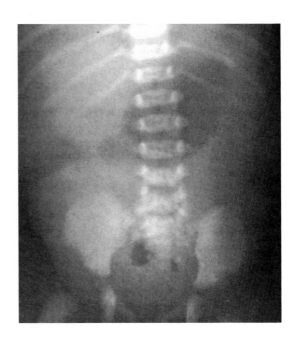

FIGURE 15-11
Annular pancreas. The small amount of gas distal to the obstruction indicates that it is not a complete atresia. (From Gore RM, Levine MS, Laufer I, eds. *Textbook of gastrointestinal radiology.* Philadelphia: WB Saunders, 1994, with permission.)

Suggested Reading
Free EA. Duodenal obstruction in the newborn due to annular pancreas. *AJR* 1968;103:321.

Intestinal Atresia

KEY FACTS

- Congenital jejunal and ileal atresia are major causes of mechanical small bowel obstruction in infants and young children
- Meconium peritonitis is a complication

JEJUNAL ATRESIA

KEY FACTS

- Triple-bubble sign (stomach, duodenum, proximal jejunum)

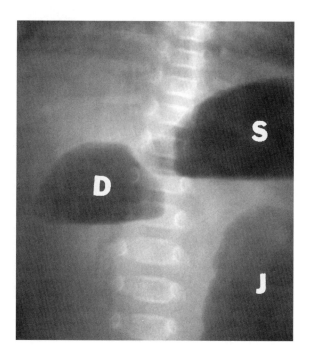

FIGURE 15-12
Jejunal atresia (triple-bubble sign). *S*, stomach; *D*, duodenum; *J*, jejunum.

ILEAL ATRESIA

KEY FACTS

- Diffusely dilated intestinal loops (more than three bubbles)
- May be difficult to determine whether the dilated intestinal loops seen on plain radiographs represent large or small bowel (barium enema may be required to make this differentiation)
- Ribbon-like microcolon in low ileal atresia (since little or no small bowel contents have reached the colon during fetal life)

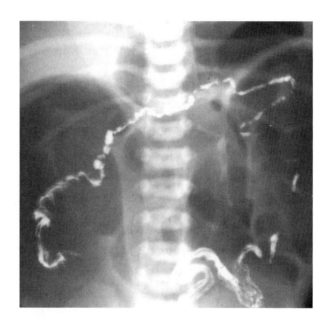

FIGURE 15-13
Ileal atresia with microcolon. Thin, ribbon-like colon in this infant with hugely distended loops of small bowel extending to the point of obstruction in the lower ileum.

Suggested Reading
Louw JH. Jejunoileal atresia and stenosis. *J Pediatr Surg* 1966;1:8.

Amyloidosis of the Small Bowel

KEY FACTS

- Deposition of amorphous eosinophilic amyloid in and around the walls of small blood vessels and between muscle fibers of the small bowel
- Usually secondary to some chronic inflammatory or necrotizing process (e.g., tuberculosis, rheumatoid arthritis, osteomyelitis, ulcerative colitis, malignant neoplasm) or multiple myeloma
- Small intestinal involvement occurs in at least 70% of cases of generalized amyloidosis
- Radiographic findings include:
  a. generalized irregular thickening of small bowel folds
  b. small bowel dilatation (due to ischemic alteration of motility)
  c. multiple nodular filling defects (uncommon)

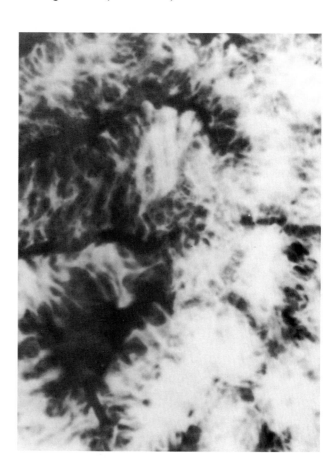

FIGURE 15-14
Amyloidosis. Irregular thickening of small bowel folds.

Suggested Reading

Carlson HC, Breen JF. Amyloidosis and plasma cell dyscrasias: gastrointestinal involvement. *Semin Roentgenol* 1986;21:128.

Brunner's Gland Hyperplasia

KEY FACTS

- Reactive response of the duodenal mucosa to peptic ulcer disease (alkaline secretion of Brunner's glands is rich in mucus and bicarbonate, which protects the sensitive duodenal mucosa from erosion by stomach acid)
- Multiple nodular filling defects, primarily in the duodenal bulb and the proximal half of the second portion
- May present as a large discrete filling defect (Brunner's gland "adenoma")

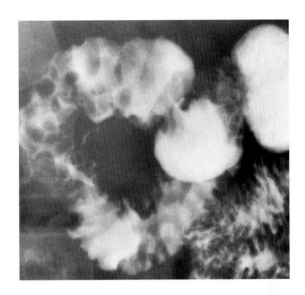

FIGURE 15-15

Brunner's gland hyperplasia. Multiple nodules produce a cobblestone appearance involving the duodenal bulb and sweep.

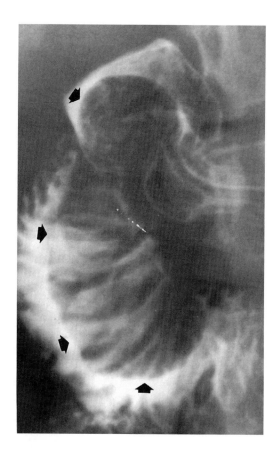

FIGURE 15-16
Brunner's gland adenoma. Large filling
defect *(arrows)* involving the duodenal
bulb and sweep.

Suggested Reading

Merine D, Jones B, Ghahremani GG, et al. Hyperplasia of Brunner glands: the spectrum of its
radiographic manifestations. *Gastrointest Radiol* 1991;16:104.

Chronic Idiopathic Intestinal Pseudo-obstruction

KEY FACTS

- Episodic signs and symptoms of mechanical small bowel obstruction without any organic lesion
- Unclear etiology, though probably related to various abnormalities of smooth muscle and the intramural nerve plexuses
- Recognition of this condition may prevent unnecessary laparotomies
- Radiographic pattern of small bowel dilatation identical to that of mechanical obstruction

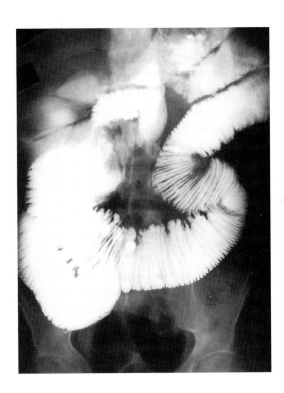

FIGURE 15-17

Chronic idiopathic pseudo-obstruction. Diffuse small bowel dilatation simulating mechanical small bowel obstruction. (From Maldonado JE, Gregg JA, Green PA, et al. Chronic idiopathic pseudo-obstruction. *Am J Med* 1970;49:203, with permission.)

Suggested Reading

Maldonado JE, Gregg JA, Green PA, et al. Chronic idiopathic pseudo-obstruction. *Am J Med* 1970;49:203.

Small Bowel Diverticula

DUODENAL DIVERTICULUM

KEY FACTS

- Incidental finding in 5% of barium examinations (often multiple)
- Most commonly found along the medial border of the descending duodenum in the periampullary region
- Anomalous insertion of the common bile duct and pancreatic duct into a duodenal diverticulum can promote retrograde inflammation
- Smooth rounded shape with normal mucosal folds
- Generally changes configuration during the study

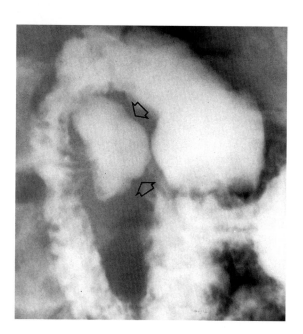

FIGURE 15-18
Duodenal diverticulum *(arrows)*.

Suggested Reading

Nelson JA, Burhenne HJ. Anomalous biliary and pancreatic duct insertion into duodenal diverticula. *Radiology* 1976;120:49.

INTRALUMINAL DUODENAL DIVERTICULUM

KEY FACTS

- Finger-like sac (windsock appearance) that is separated from contrast material in the duodenal lumen by a lucent band representing the diverticular wall (halo sign)
- Related to forward pressure by food and strong peristaltic activity on a thin, incomplete congenital duodenal web originating near the papilla of Vater

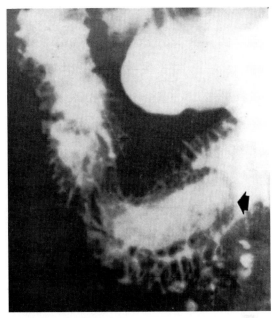

A

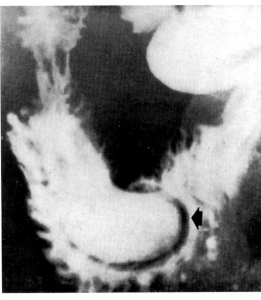

FIGURE 15-19
Intraluminal duodenal diverticulum. "Halo" sign *(arrow)* seen with the diverticulum partially (**A**) and completely (**B**) filled with barium. (From Laudan JCH, Norton GI. Intraluminal duodenal diverticulum. *AJR* 1963;90:756, with permission.)

B

Suggested Reading
Laudan JCH, Norton GI. Intraluminal duodenal diverticulum. *AJR* 1963;90:756.

JEJUNAL DIVERTICULUM

KEY FACTS

- Usually multiple and with wider necks than colonic diverticula
- May produce the blind loop system with bacterial overgrowth and folic acid deficiency
- A major cause of pneumoperitoneum without peritonitis or surgery

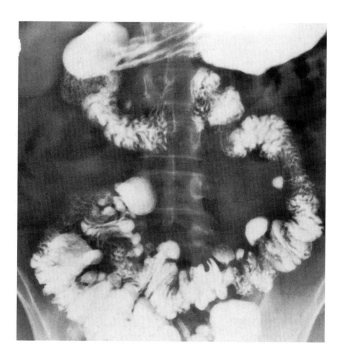

FIGURE 15-20
Jejunal diverticulosis.

Suggested Reading

Dunn V, Nelson JA. Jejunal diverticulosis and chronic pneumoperitoneum. *Gastrointest Radiol* 1979;4:165.

MECKEL'S DIVERTICULUM

KEY FACTS

- Most frequent congenital anomaly of the intestinal tract (2% to 3% of the population)
- Blind outpouching representing the rudimentary omphalomesenteric duct (embryonic communication between the gut and the yolk sac) that is normally obliterated by the fifth embryonic week
- Arises on the antimesenteric side of the ileum within 100 cm of the ileocecal valve
- May be inflamed and simulate acute appendicitis, or may contain heterotopic gastric mucosa (seen on a technetium scan)

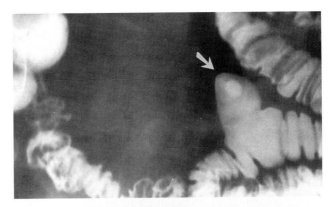

FIGURE 15-21
Meckel's diverticulum. Note the small diverticulum (area of increased density) arising from it.

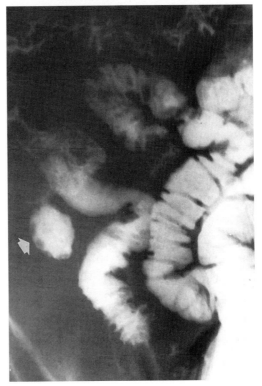

FIGURE 15-22
Meckel's diverticulum. Ectopic gastric mucosa appears as multiple filling defects *(arrow)* within the diverticulum.

Suggested Reading

Miller KB, Naimark A, O'Connor JF, et al. Unusual roentgenologic manifestations of Meckel's diverticulum. *Gastrointest Radiol* 1981;6:209.

ILEAL DIVERTICULUM

KEY FACTS

- Least common of the small bowel diverticula
- Small, often multiple, and situated in the terminal portion near the ileocecal valve
- Ileal diverticulitis (rare) may present clinical symptoms indistinguishable from acute appendicitis

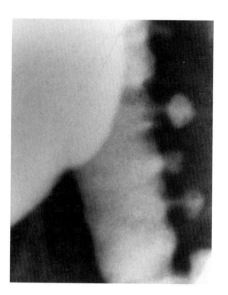

FIGURE 15-23

Ileal diverticula. These diverticula are located near the ileocecal valve, unlike Meckel's diverticula, which are situated more proximally.

Suggested Reading

Maglinte DDT, Chernish SM, DeWeese R, et al. Acquired jejunoileal diverticular disease: subject review. *Radiology* 1986;158:577.

PSEUDODIVERTICULA

KEY FACTS

- In *scleroderma*, large sacculations involving the antimesenteric border with squared, broad bases (result from smooth muscle atrophy and fibrosis)
- In *Crohn's disease*, pseudodiverticula are associated with strictures and characteristic mucosal changes
- In *lymphoma*, there is fusiform aneurysmal dilatation of the bowel that is not restricted to one wall (see Fig. 14-7)

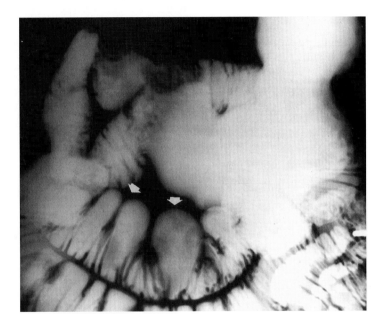

FIGURE 15-24 Pseudodiverticula (scleroderma). Wide-mouthed sacculations with squared broad bases *(arrows)*.

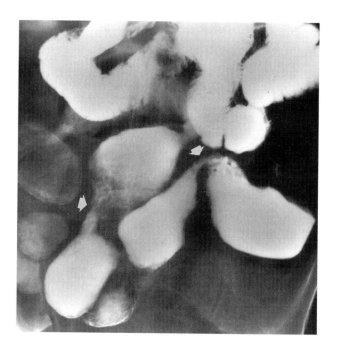

FIGURE 15-25
Pseudodiverticula (Crohn's disease). The apparent diverticula actually reflect normal bowel between tightly strictured areas *(arrows)*.

Suggested Reading

Oueloz JM, Woloshin HJ. Sacculation of the small intestine in scleroderma. *Radiology* 1972; 105:513.

Hemorrhage into Small Bowel Wall

KEY FACTS

- Major causes include anticoagulant therapy, hemophilia, vasculitis, idiopathic thrombocytopenic purpura, and coagulation defects secondary to malignant or other diseases
- Uniform regular thickening of small bowel folds ("stack of coins" appearance)
- Concomitant bleeding into the mesentery often results in an intramural or extrinsic mass and separation and uncoiling of bowel loops

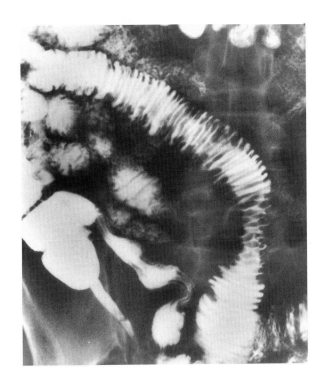

FIGURE 15-26
Hemorrhage into the bowel wall and mesentery. Regular thickening of folds and separation and uncoiling of bowel loops due to Coumadin overdose.

Suggested Reading
Schwartz S, Boley S, Schultz L, et al. A survey of vascular diseases of the small intestine. *Semin Roentgenol* 1966;1:178.

Intestinal Edema

KEY FACTS

- Major causes include:
  a. hypoproteinemia (cirrhosis, renal failure) with decreased oncotic pressure
  b. fluid overload
  c. increased venous pressure (congestive failure, portal hypertension)
  d. lymphatic blockage
- Uniform regular thickening of small bowel folds

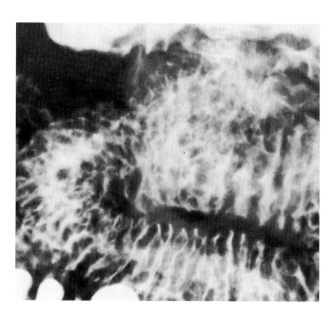

FIGURE 15-27
Intestinal edema (hypoproteinemia). Regular thickening of small bowel folds in a patient with cirrhosis.

Suggested Reading

Marshak RH, Khilnani MT, Eliasoph J, et al. Intestinal edema. *AJR* 1967;101:379.

Intestinal Lymphangiectasia

KEY FACTS

- Gross dilatation of the lymphatics in the mucosa and submucosa of the small bowel
- *Primary* form represents a congenital mechanical block to lymphatic outflow
- *Secondary* form is a complication of inflammatory or neoplastic lymphadenopathy
- Regular thickening of small bowel folds caused by a combination of lymphatic dilatation and intestinal edema (due to lymphatic obstruction or severe protein loss)

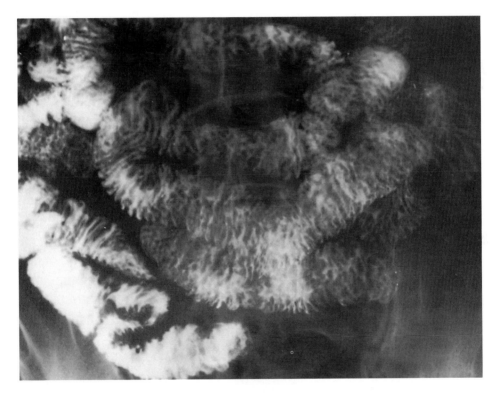

FIGURE 15-28   Intestinal lymphangiectasia. Regular thickening of small bowel folds secondary to lymphatic obstruction due to infiltration of the bowel wall and mesentery by metastatic carcinoma.

Suggested Reading
Shimkin PM, Waldmann TA, Krugman RL. Intestinal lymphangiectasia. *AJR* 1970;110:827.

Intussusception

KEY FACTS

- Invagination or prolapse of a segment of bowel (intussusceptum) into the lumen of adjacent intestine (intussuscipiens) due to peristalsis
- Major cause of small bowel obstruction in children (much less common in adults)
- In *adults*, the leading edge of an intussusception (usually a pedunculated polypoid tumor) can be demonstrated in 80% of cases
- In *children*, intussusception is most common in the region of the ileocecal valve and frequently no anatomic etiology is apparent
- Classic coiled-spring appearance (barium trapped between the intussusceptum and the surrounding portions of bowel)
- On CT, three concentric rings
  - a. central ring—lumen and wall of intussusceptum
  - b. middle ring—crescent of mesenteric fat
  - c. outer ring—returning intussusceptum and intussuscipiens
- On ultrasound, "doughnut" sign on transverse sections and "pseudokidney" sign on longitudinal scans

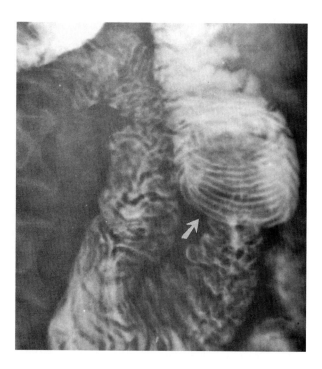

FIGURE 15-29
Jejunojejunal intussusception.
Classic coiled-spring appearance
(arrow).

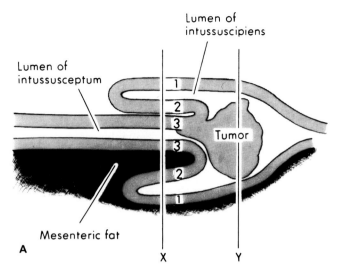

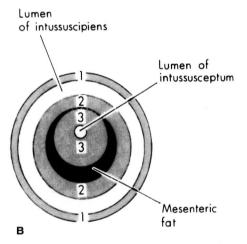

FIGURE 15-30
CT of intussusception.
A: Diagram of a longitudinal section through an intussusception. *1*, wall of intussuscipiens; *2, 3*, folded layers of bowel wall that constitute the intussusceptum. Note how invaginated mesenteric fat is attached to one side of the intussusceptum and separates the wall of the intussusceptum into two individual layers. **B:** Diagram of the cross section of the intussusception at level *X* in **A.** Note the eccentric lumen of the intussusceptum. Where mesenteric fat is present, three distinct layers (1,2,3) can be seen. Only two layers are visible where there is no mesenteric fat, because layers 2 and 3 cannot be distinguished. **C:** In this patient with an ileocolic intussusception, a cross-sectional view shows contrast material in the ascending colon *(white arrowheads)* surrounding the intussuscepted ileum and associated mesenteric fat. A tiny amount of contrast material is seen in the ileal lumen *(black arrowhead)*. Lymphoma of the ileum formed the leading mass. (From Mauro MA, Koehler RE. Alimentary tract. In: Lee JKT, Sagel SS, Stanley RJ, eds. *Computed body tomography.* New York: Raven Press, 1983, with permission.)

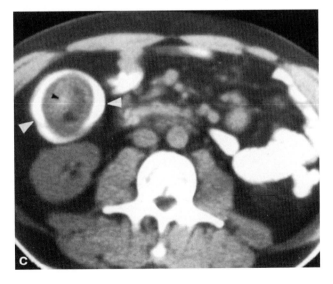

Suggested Reading
Agha FP. Intussusception in adults. *AJR* 1986;146:527.

Intramural Duodenal Hematoma

KEY FACTS

- Most commonly a complication of blunt trauma to the abdomen (since the duodenum is the most fixed portion of the small bowel)
- 80% of reported cases have been in children or young adults, and child abuse is a major cause in infants and young children
- May be secondary to anticoagulant therapy or an abnormal bleeding diathesis
- Appears radiographically as a sharply defined, tumor-like intramural mass that narrows or even completely obstructs the duodenal lumen

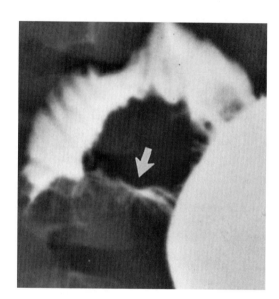

FIGURE 15-31

Intramural duodenal hematoma. High-grade stenotic lesion *(arrow)* in a young child who had been kicked in the abdomen by his father.

Suggested Reading
Radin DR. Intramural and intraperitoneal hemorrhage due to duodenal ulcer. *AJR* 1991;157:45.

Lactase Deficiency

KEY FACTS

- Most common of the disaccharidase-deficiency syndromes, in which an isolated enzyme defect prevents the proper hydrolysis and absorption of the major sugar in milk products
- High incidence (>75% of adults) in African-Americans, Chinese, and Mexicans
- Patients experience abdominal discomfort, cramps, and watery diarrhea 30 minutes to several hours after ingesting milk or milk products
- Radiographic appearance of generalized small bowel dilatation with dilution of barium, rapid transit time, and reproduction of symptoms after the oral administration of lactose

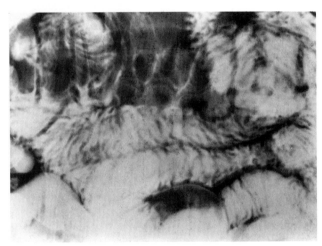

A

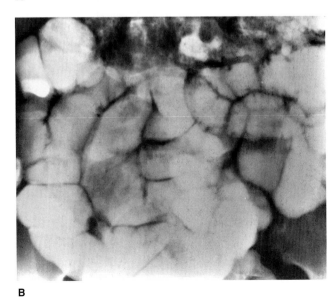

FIGURE 15-32
Lactase deficiency.
A: Normal conventional small bowel examination.
B: After the addition of 50 g of lactose to the barium mixture, there is marked dilatation of the small bowel with dilution of barium, rapid transit, and reproduction of symptoms.

B

Suggested Reading

Preger L, Amberg JR. Sweet diarrhea: roentgen diagnosis of disaccharidase deficiency. *AJR* 1967;101:287.

Macroglobulinemia (Waldenstrom's Disease)

KEY FACTS

- Plasma cell dyscrasia involving those cells that synthesize macroglobulins (IgM)
- Insidious onset in late adult life with anemia, bleeding, lymphadenopathy, and hepatosplenomegaly
- Lacteals and lamina propria of small bowel villi are filled with macroglobulin proteinaceous material
- Characteristic sand-like pattern of innumerable fine punctate lucencies in the barium column

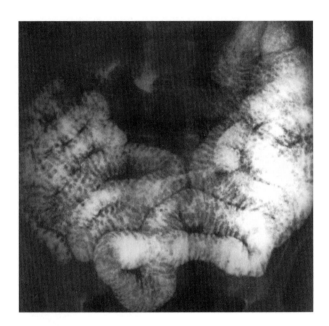

FIGURE 15-33
Macroglobulinemia
(Waldenstrom's disease).

Suggested Reading

Bedine MS, Yardley JH, Elliott HL, et al. Intestinal involvement in Waldenstrom's macroglobulinemia. *Gastroenterology* 1973;65:308.

Mastocytosis

KEY FACTS

- Systemic mast cell proliferation in the reticuloendothelial system and skin (urticaria pigmentosa)
- High incidence of peptic ulcers, pruritus, flushing, tachycardia, asthma, and headaches due to the episodic release of histamine from mast cells
- Generalized irregular, distorted, thickened folds throughout the small bowel
- Other characteristic findings include hepatosplenomegaly, lymphadenopathy, and sclerotic bone lesions

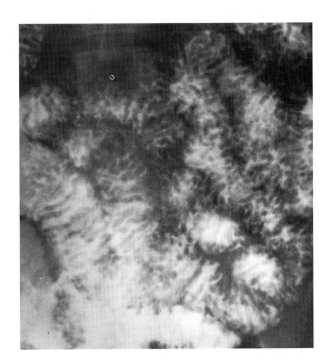

FIGURE 15-34
Mastocytosis. Generalized irregular, distorted small bowel folds.

Suggested Reading

Clemett AR, Fishbone G, Levine RJ, et al. Gastrointestinal lesions in mastocytosis. *AJR* 1968;103:405.

Meconium Peritonitis

KEY FACTS

- Complication of high-grade small bowel obstruction *in utero* in which a proximal perforation permits meconium to pass into the peritoneal cavity and incite an inflammatory response
- Often produces multiple small flecks of calcification scattered widely throughout the abdomen in a newborn
- May be larger aggregates of calcification along the inferior surface of the liver, in the flanks, or extending along the processus vaginalis to the scrotum
- Fetal ultrasound findings include:
  a. fetal ascites that may have echogenic debris
  b. echogenicity along the peritoneal surfaces
  c. abnormal cystic abdominal masses
  d. dilated bowel with thickened walls

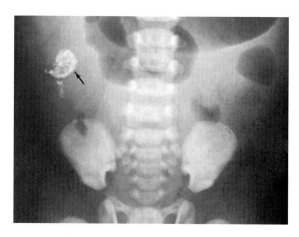

FIGURE 15-35 Meconium peritonitis. Plain abdominal radiograph in an 18-day-old infant in whom signs of intestinal obstruction developed weeks after birth shows the calciferous meconium collected in a single large cluster *(arrow)* in the right side of the abdomen. The gas column in the alimentary tract is cut off in a fashion indicative of complete obstruction high in the small intestine. (From Silverman SN. *Caffey's pediatric x-ray imaging.* Chicago: Year Book, 1985, with permission.)

FIGURE 15-36

Meconium peritonitis. Longitudinal sonogram reveals a peritoneal collection of meconium *(arrows)* anterior to the echogenic neonatal kidney *(K)*. The meconium is less echogenic than the solid structures, but contains more echoes than a simple transudative ascites. *H,* superior; *F,* inferior (From Gore RM, Levine MS, Laufer I, eds. *Textbook of gastrointestinal radiology.* Philadelphia: WB Saunders, 1994, with permission.)

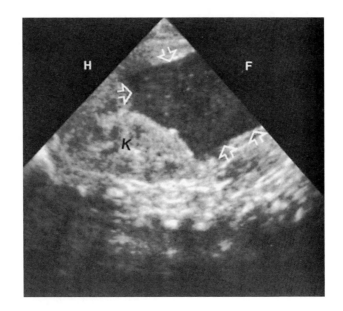

Suggested Reading

Leonidas J, Berdon WE, Baker DH, et al. Meconium ileus and its complications. *AJR* 1970; 108:598.

Meconium Ileus

KEY FACTS

- Low small bowel obstruction secondary to inspissated meconium that impacts in the distal ileum
- Caused by thick and sticky meconium (due to the absence of normal pancreatic and intestinal gland secretions during fetal life) that cannot be readily propelled through the bowel
- Frequent association with cystic fibrosis
- Bubbly or frothy appearance of intestinal contents on plain films
- Microcolon (since it has not been used during fetal life)

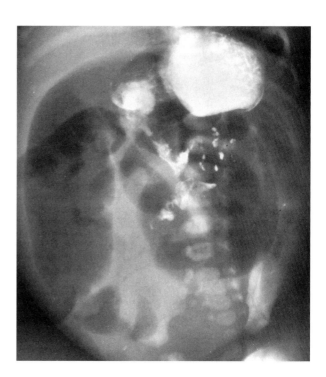

FIGURE 15-37
Meconium ileus.

Suggested Reading

Leonidas J, Berdon WE, Baker DH, et al. Meconium ileus and its complications. *AJR* 1970; 108:598.

Prolapsed Antral Mucosa

KEY FACTS

- Prolapse of redundant antral folds into the duodenal bulb due to active peristalsis
- As the peristaltic wave relaxes, the mucosal folds tend to return to the antrum and the defect at the base of the bulb diminishes or completely disappears
- Mucosal folds in the prepyloric area of the stomach usually can be traced through the pylorus to the base of the bulb, where they become continuous with the prolapsed mass

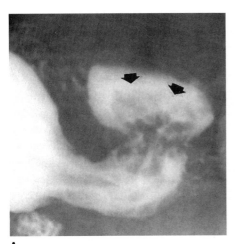
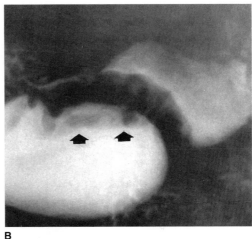

A   B

FIGURE 15-38   Prolapsed antral mucosa. **A:** Appearance of a mass *(arrows)* in the duodenal bulb. **B:** With reduction of the prolapse, the mass in the base of the bulb disappears and the redundant antral folds become evident *(arrows)*.

Suggested Reading

Eisenberg RL. *Gastrointestinal radiology: a pattern approach.* Philadelphia: Lippincott–Raven Publishers, 1996.

Nodular Lymphoid Hyperplasia

KEY FACTS

- In adults, almost invariably associated with late-onset immunoglobulin deficiency (increased susceptibility to respiratory and other infections)
- *Giardia lamblia* infection can be demonstrated in up to 90% of patients
- Diarrhea and malabsorption are frequent complaints
- Sand-like pattern of innumerable filling defects that primarily involves the jejunum but can be distributed uniformly throughout the entire small bowel
- In children and young adults, the presence of multiple small symmetric nodules of lymphoid hyperplasia in the terminal ileum is a normal finding (no immune deficiency)

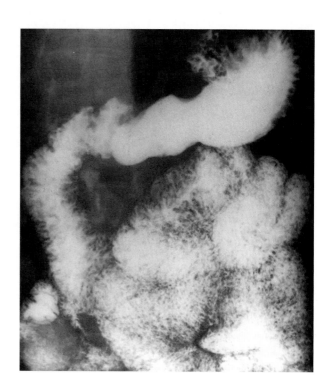

FIGURE 15-39

Nodular lymphoid hyperplasia. Sand-like pattern of innumerable tiny polypoid masses that are uniformly distributed throughout the involved segments of small bowel.

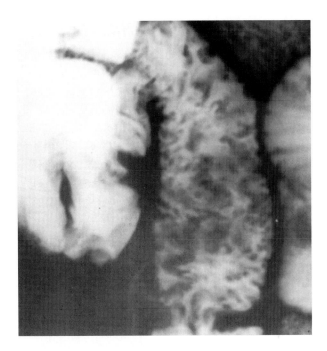

FIGURE 15-40

Normal terminal ileum in an adolescent. Multiple small nodules represent normal prominence of lymphoid follicles.

Suggested Reading

Ament ME, Rubin CE. Relation of giardiasis to abnormal intestinal structure and function in gastrointestinal immunodeficiency syndromes. *Gastroenterology* 1972;62:216.

Radiation Enteritis

KEY FACTS

- Complication of large-dose radiation therapy to adjacent organs
- Small bowel is the most radiosensitive organ in the abdomen, but natural peristalsis serves as a protective mechanism (unless previous abdominal surgery has adhesively anchored bowel loops)
- Thickening of the bowel wall (submucosal edema and fibrosis) leads to separation of adjacent small bowel loops
- Progressive fibrosis results in tapered strictures, which commonly involve long segments
- Fistulas to the vagina or other organs may occur
- On CT, bowel wall thickening, increased density of the mesentery, and fixation of bowel loops

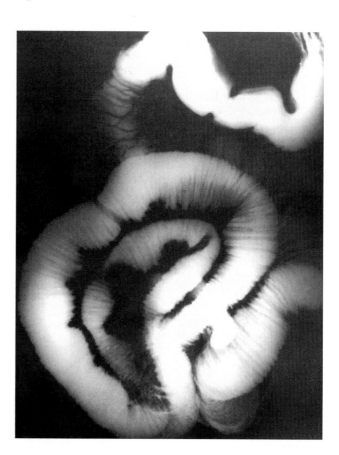

FIGURE 15-41

Radiation enteritis. Thickening of the bowel wall and multiple nodular masses cause separation of small bowel loops. The patient had received 7,000 rad (70 Gy) for treatment of metastatic carcinoma of the cervix.

Suggested Reading

Rogers LF, Goldstein HM. Roentgen manifestations of radiation injury to the gastrointestinal tract. *Gastrointest Radiol* 1977;2:281.

Part E
COLON

16 Inflammatory/Infectious Colitides

Ulcerative Colitis

KEY FACTS

- Ulcerative inflammation that primarily involves the rectum (spared in 5% of cases) and then progresses proximally (may be pancolitis)
- "Backwash ileitis" develops in 10% to 25% of cases
- The inflammatory changes generally are confined to the mucosa
- Unknown etiology, though appears to represent some type of hypersensitivity or autoimmune response
- Typically produces relatively mild abdominal cramps and bloody diarrhea with alternating periods of remission and exacerbation
- In less than 10%, acute fulminant process with systemic toxicity, severe diarrhea, and electrolyte depletion
- Complications include toxic megacolon, stricture formation, perforation, and a significantly increased risk of developing colon carcinoma
- Extracolonic manifestations include spondylitis, peripheral arthritis, iritis, skin disorders (erythema nodosum, pyoderma gangrenosum), and various liver abnormalities
- Radiographic findings include:
  a. fine mucosal granularity (initial appearance)
  b. stippled pattern due to superficial ulcerations
  c. collar-button ulcers
  d. pseudopolyposis (scattered islands of hyperplastic inflamed mucosa between interlacing areas of ulceration
  e. progressive shortening and rigidity of the colon ("lead pipe"), which represents fibrotic reaction and muscular hypertrophy and spasm in chronic disease
  f. benign colonic stricture with concentric lumen, smooth contours, and pliable tapering margins (may be indistinguishable from carcinoma in patients with this disease)
  g. toxic megacolon
- On CT, inhomogeneous thickening of the bowel wall with areas of low attenuation

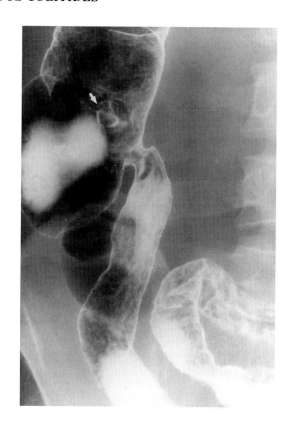

FIGURE 16-1

Backwash ileitis in ulcerative colitis. The terminal ileum and cecum have lost their normal fold pattern, and the mucosa appears coarsely granular. Note the patulous ileocecal valve and the single large inflammatory polyp *(arrow)*. (From Caroline DF, Evers K. Colitis: radiographic features and differentiation of idiopathic inflammatory bowel disease. *Radiol Clin North Am* 1987;25:47, with permission.)

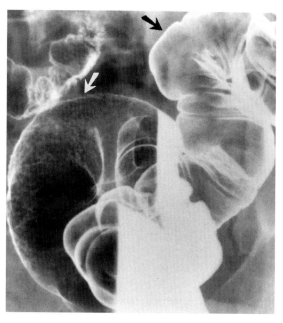

FIGURE 16-2

Ulcerative colitis. The distal rectosigmoid mucosa *(white arrow)* has a finely granular appearance when compared with the normal-appearing mucosa *(black arrow)* in the uninvolved more proximal colon.

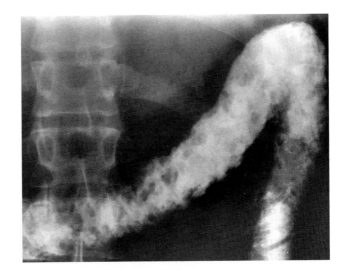

FIGURE 16-3
Ulcerative colitis. Irregular
pseudopolyps associated with
a severe ulcerating process.

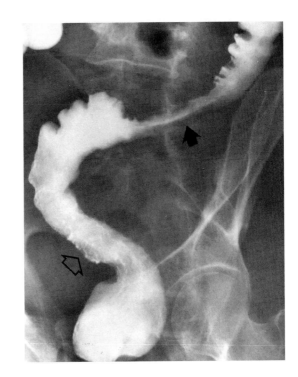

FIGURE 16-4
Chronic ulcerative colitis. Benign
stricture in the sigmoid colon *(solid
arrow)*. Note the ulcerative changes in
the upper rectum and proximal
sigmoid colon *(open arrow)*.

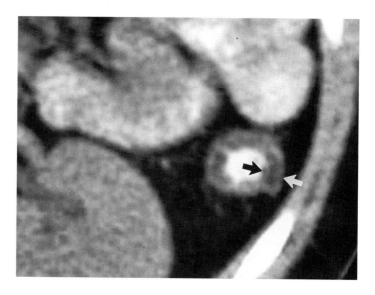

FIGURE 16-5   Ulcerative colitis. CT scan at the level of the lower pole of the left kidney shows inhomogeneous thickening of the descending colon with several areas of decreased attenuation *(arrows)*. (From Gore RM, Marn CS, Kirby DF, et al. CT findings in ulcerative, granulomatous, and indeterminate colitis. *AJR* 1984;143:279, with permission.)

Suggested Readings

Caroline DF, Evers K. Colitis: radiographic features and differentiation of idiopathic inflammatory bowel disease. *Radiol Clin North Am* 1987:25:47.

Gore RM, Marn CS, Kirby DF, et al. CT findings in ulcerative, granulomatous, and indeterminate colitis. *AJR* 1984;143:279.

Crohn's Colitis

KEY FACTS

- Diffuse chronic transmural inflammatory process (identical to the same pathologic process involving the small bowel)
- Clinical symptoms include diarrhea (more distressing and intense than in ulcerative colitis, but rarely gross blood), crampy and colicky abdominal pain, insidious weight loss, perianal or perirectal abnormalities (fissures, hemorrhoids, abscesses) and enterocutaneous fistulas
- Extra-intestinal manifestations include large joint migratory polyarthritis, ankylosing spondylitis, sclerosing cholangitis, and renal oxalate stones
- Primarily affects the proximal colon, with a high incidence of terminal ileal involvement
- Features that suggest Crohn's disease rather than ulcerative colitis include:
  a. noncontinuous skip lesions, which are common
  b. aphthous ulcers on a background of normal mucosa (not the granular pattern of ulcerative colitis)
  c. random and asymmetric distribution of deep irregular ulcers (not uniform and monotonous as in ulcerative colitis)
  d. cobblestone appearance (due to transverse and longitudinal ulcerations separated by pseudopolypoid islands of thickened mucosa and submucosa)
  e. spontaneous fistulas and sinus tracts
  f. severe anal and perianal disease
- CT findings suggesting Crohn's disease include:
  a. bowel wall is generally thicker and has more homogeneous attenuation
  b. fibro-fatty proliferation ("creeping fat") of the mesentery
  c. mesenteric adenopathy and abscesses
  d. fistulas
  e. perirectal/perianal abnormalities

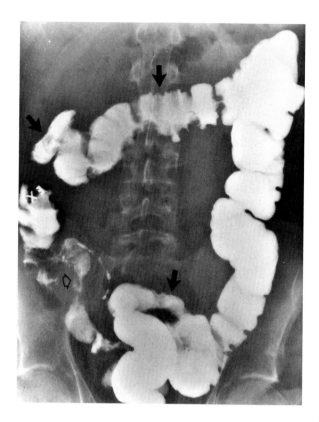

FIGURE 16-6

Crohn's colitis (skip lesions). Areas of involved colon in the ascending, transverse, and sigmoid regions *(solid arrows)* are separated by normal appearing segments. Note the inflammatory changes affecting the distal ileum *(open arrow)*.

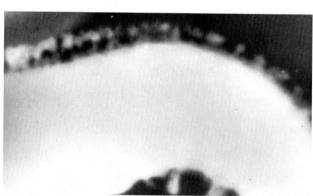

FIGURE 16-7

Crohn's colitis. "Collar-button" ulcers distributed asymmetrically around the circumference of the bowel.

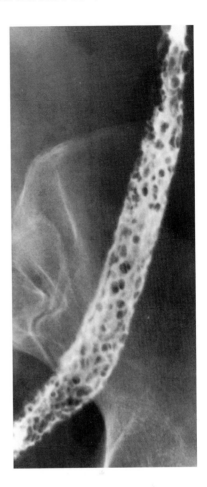

FIGURE 16-8

Crohn's disease. Coarsely nodular "cobblestone" appearance produced by swollen and edematous mucosa surrounded by long, deep, linear ulcers and transverse fissures.

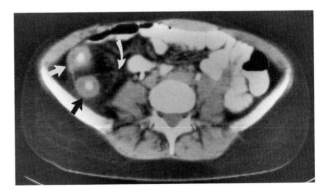

FIGURE 16-9   Crohn's disease. CT scan shows homogeneous thickening of the ascending colon *(straight white arrow)* and distal ileum *(black arrow).* Note the abnormal mesenteric fat *(curved arrow)* and separation of abnormal segments from other small bowel loops. The descending colon has normal mural thickness. (From Gore RM, Marn CS, Kirby DF, et al. CT findings in ulcerative, granulomatous, and indeterminate colitis. *AJR* 1984;143:279, with permission.)

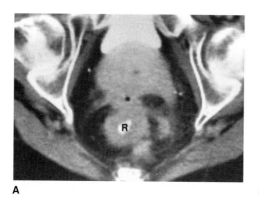
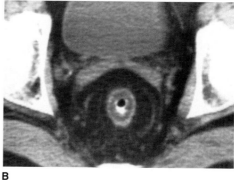

A   B

FIGURE 16-10   Comparison of CT appearance of Crohn's and ulcerative colitis. **A:** In Crohn's colitis, there is marked homogeneous thickening of the rectum *(R)*, with abnormal soft-tissue densities in the left perirectal space. **B:** In ulcerative colitis, the rectum produces a "target" appearance consisting of contrast- or air-filled lumen surrounded by a ring of soft-tissue density, which in turn is surrounded by a ring of decreased attenuation and finally encompassed by a ring of soft-tissue density. Scattered abnormal streaky densities can be seen in the presacral fat. (From Gore RM, Marn CS, Kirby DF, et al. CT findings in ulcerative, granulomatous, and indeterminate colitis. *AJR* 1984;143:279, with permission.)

Suggested Readings

Caroline DF, Evers K. Colitis: radiographic features and differentiation of idiopathic inflammatory bowel disease. *Radiol Clin North Am* 1987;25:47.

Gore RM, Marn CS, Kirby DF, et al. CT findings in ulcerative, granulomatous, and indeterminate colitis. *AJR* 1984;143:279.

Ischemic Colitis

KEY FACTS

- Abrupt onset of lower abdominal pain and rectal bleeding (may also be abdominal pain and diarrhea)
- Usually occurs in patients of age >50 who have a history of prior cardiovascular disease
- Predisposing factors include volvulus, carcinoma, bleeding disorders, and contraceptive pills
- Particularly vulnerable areas are the "watershed" regions between two adjacent major arterial supplies (splenic flexure and sigmoid)
- The rectum is rarely involved because of its excellent collateral blood supply
- Usually involves a relatively short segment (pancolitis can occur) and returns to a normal appearance
- Short strictures that infrequently develop with healing may mimic annular carcinoma
- Radiographic findings include:
  a. fine superficial ulcerations (initially)
  b. deep penetrating ulcers with pseudopolyposis
  c. thumbprinting (finger-like marginal indentations along the wall of the colon)
- On CT, symmetric bowel wall thickening, sometimes with a target or double-halo pattern and polypoid defects associated with thumbprinting

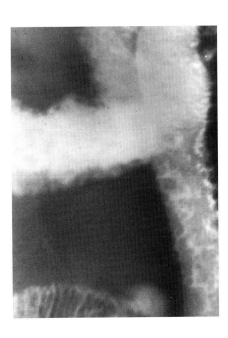

FIGURE 16-11
Ischemic colitis. Superficial ulcers and inflammatory edema produce a serrated outer margin of the barium-filled colon simulating ulcerative colitis.

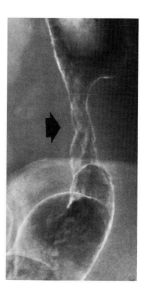

FIGURE 16-12

Ischemic colitis. Stricture in the descending colon *(arrow)* following healing of the ischemic episode. (From Eisenberg RL, Montgomery CK, Margulis AR. Colitis in the elderly: ischemic colitis mimicking ulcerative and granulomatous colitis. *AJR* 1979;133:1113, with permission.)

Suggested Reading

Iida M, Matsui T, Fuchigami T, et al. Ischemic colitis: serial changes on double-contrast barium enema examination. *Radiology* 1986;159:337.

Amebic Colitis

KEY FACTS

- Primary infection of the colon by the protozoan *Entamoeba histolytica*, which is acquired by the ingestion of food or water contaminated by amebic cysts
- Patient is asymptomatic (carrier state) until the protozoan actually invades the wall of the colon and incites an inflammatory reaction
- Clinical symptoms range from mild abdominal discomfort and intermittent diarrhea to acute attacks of frequent diarrhea, blood and mucus in the stools, and cramping abdominal pain that tends to be located in the right lower quadrant
- Primarily involves the cecum and right colon (terminal ileum virtually never involved, unlike Crohn's disease and tuberculosis)
- Radiographic findings include
  a. superficial ulcerations (initially)
  b. deep penetrating ulcers that may produce a bizarre appearance
  c. coned cecum (due to concentric fibrotic narrowing)
  d. fixation of thickened ileocecal valve in an open position (with reflux)
  e. annular constriction (ameboma) simulating malignancy
- Factors favoring ameboma rather than malignancy include multiplicity, longer length and pliability of the lesion, and rapid improvement on antiamebic therapy

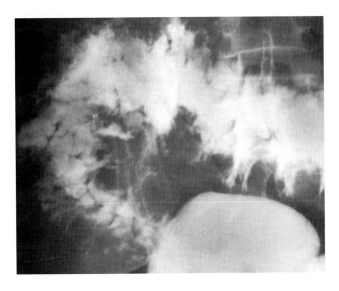

FIGURE 16-13   Amebic colitis. Deep penetrating ulcers produce a bizarre appearance.

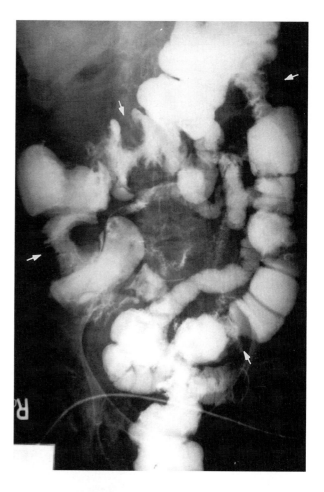

FIGURE 16-14

Ameboma. Multiple classic "apple-core" lesions *(arrows)* with irregular mucosa and overhanging edges. (From Messersmith RN, Chase GJ. Amebiasis presenting as multiple apple-core lesions. *Am J Gastroenterol* 1984;79:238, with permission.)

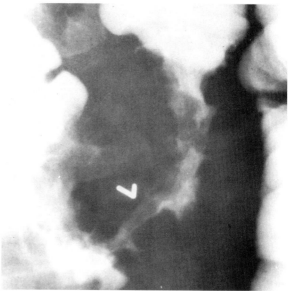

FIGURE 16-15

Ameboma. The relatively long length of this irregular constricting lesion of the transverse colon tends to favor an inflammatory etiology.

Suggested Reading

Messersmith RN, Chase GJ. Amebiasis presenting as multiple apple-core lesions. *Am J Gastroenterol* 1984;79:238.

Lymphogranuloma Venereum

KEY FACTS

- Venereal disease caused by *Chlamydia trachomatis* that is especially common in the tropics
- Primarily involves the rectum (occasionally extends proximally to the sigmoid and descending colon)
- Radiographic hallmark is a rectal stricture beginning just above the anus (varies from a short isolated narrowing to a long stenotic segment with multiple deep ulcers)
- Fistulas and sinus tracts often occur

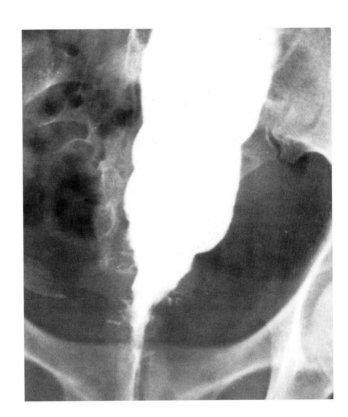

FIGURE 16-16

Lymphogranuloma venereum. Long rectal stricture with multiple deep ulcers. (From Dreyfuss JR, Janower ML. *Radiology of the colon.* Baltimore: Williams & Wilkins, 1980.)

Suggested Reading

Cockshott WP, Middlemiss H. *Clinical radiology in the tropics.* Edinburgh: Churchill Livingstone, 1979.

Pseudomembanous Colitis

KEY FACTS

- Most commonly a complication of antibiotics or chemotherapy, probably related to overgrowth of a resistant strain of *Clostridium difficile*
- Symptoms vary from mild diarrhea to fulminant colitis with toxic megacolon and death (usually develops within 2 days to 2 weeks after therapy begins)
- Wide transverse bands of thickened colonic wall on plain films (representing edematous and distorted haustral markings)
- Barium enema (contraindicated in severe colitis) demonstrates shaggy and irregular colonic contour due to pseudomembranes (multiple flat, raised lesions) and barium filling the clefts between them
- CT shows extensive low-attenuation thickening of the colonic wall (with streaks of contrast trapped between swollen haustra projecting into the lumen)

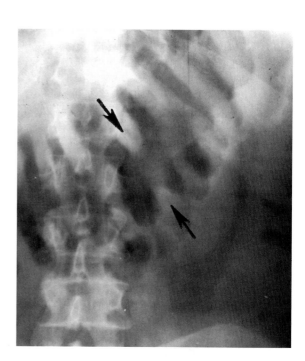

FIGURE 16-17
Pseudomembranous colitis. Plain abdominal radiograph demonstrates wide transverse bands of thickened colonic wall *(arrows)*. (From Stanley RJ, Melson GL, Tedesco FJ, et al. Plain film findings in severe pseudomembranous colitis. *Radiology* 1976;118:7, with permission.)

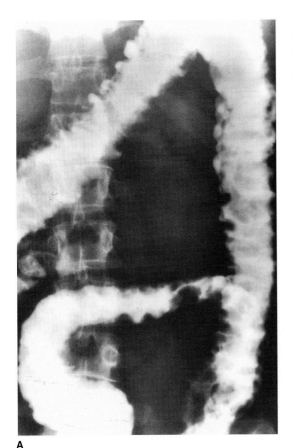

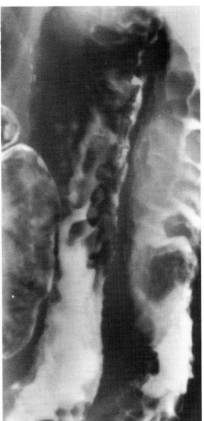

A **B**

FIGURE 16-18 Pseudomembranous colitis. **A:** Shaggy and irregular appearance of the barium column because of the pseudomembrane and superficial necrosis with mucosal ulceration. **B:** The pseudomembranes appear as multiple flat, raised lesions distributed circumferentially around the margin of the colon.

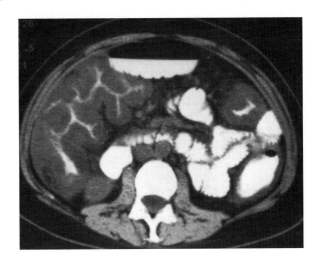

FIGURE 16-19

Pseudomembranous colitis. CT scan shows extensive low-attenuation thickening of the wall of the colon, with streaks of contrast material trapped between the swollen haustra. (From Gore RM, Levine MS, Laufer I. *Textbook of gastrointestinal radiology.* Philadelphia: WB Saunders, 1994, with permission.)

Suggested Reading

Fishman EK, Kavuru M, Jones B, et al. Pseudomembranous colitis: CT evaluation of 26 cases. *Radiology* 1991;180:57.

Cathartic Colon

KEY FACTS

- Related to prolonged use of stimulant and irritant cathartics, especially in women of middle age
- Bizarre contractions and inconstant areas of narrowing, primarily involving the right colon
- May mimic "burned-out" chronic ulcerative colitis

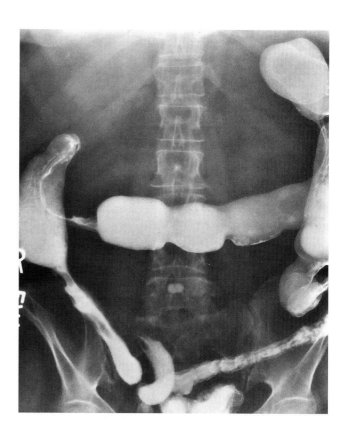

FIGURE 16-20
Cathartic colon. Bizarre contractions with irregular areas of narrowing primarily involve the right colon.

Suggested Reading

Kim SK, Gerle RD, Rozanski R. Cathartic colitis. *AJR* 1987;130:825.

Caustic Colitis

KEY FACTS

- Transient colitis that develops after a cleansing enema using potentially irritating solutions (soapsuds, detergents)
- Irritant enema tends to produce spasm of the rectosigmoid, resulting in rapid expulsion of the solution from this segment and less damage to the area
- Fluid in the proximal colon is not promptly expelled, and thus corrosive damage is most severe in this region
- Severe acute ulcerating process that may heal with fibrosis and stricture formation

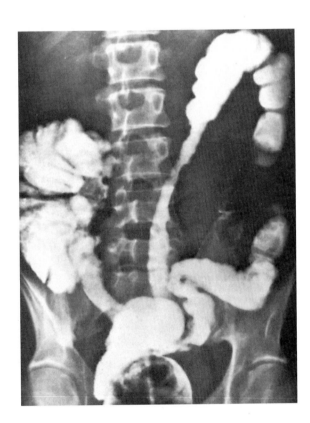

FIGURE 16-21

Caustic colitis. Diffuse ulceration and narrowing of the transverse colon. Note the mild irregularity of the rectal mucosa. (From Kim SK, Cho C., Levinsohn EM. Caustic colitis due to detergent enema. *AJR* 1980;134:397, with permission.)

Suggested Reading

Kim SK, Cho C, Levinsohn EM. Caustic colitis due to detergent enema. *AJR* 1980;134:397.

Radiation Injury of Rectum

KEY FACTS

- Usually follows pelvic irradiation for carcinoma of the cervix, endometrium, ovary, bladder or prostate
- Infrequent in patients who have received < 4,000 rad (40 Gy); substantially increased incidence with dose > 6,000 rad (60 Gy) or when a second course of radiation is given for recurrent tumor
- Radiation damage results in mucosal atrophy and fibrous tissue replacement within the bowel, leading to narrowing of the lumen
- Acutely, fine superficial (occasionally deep) ulceration simulating other ulcerating diseases of the colon
- In chronic radiation-induced colitis (developing 6 to 24 months after irradiation), a long smooth stricture of the rectum and sigmoid colon
- A short, irregular radiation-induced stricture can mimic malignancy
- CT findings include homogeneous thickening of the rectal wall, target sign, and proliferation of perirectal fat and fibrosis

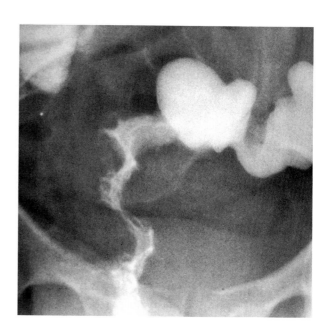

FIGURE 16-22

Radiation-induced colitis. Irregularity, spasm, and ulceration produce an appearance similar to other ulcerating diseases of the colon.

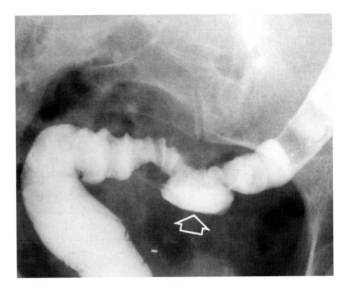

FIGURE 16-23   Radiation-induced colitis. Large, discrete penetrating ulcer *(arrow)*. (From Rogers LF, Goldstein HM. Roentgen manifestations of radiation injury to the gastrointestinal tract. *Gastrointest Radiol* 1977;2:281, with permission.)

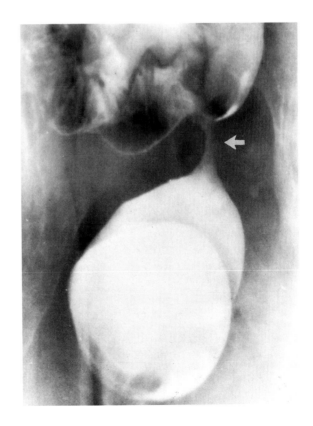

FIGURE 16-24

Radiation-induced colitis. Smooth stricture of the rectosigmoid *(arrow)* that developed 18 months after radiation therapy.

Suggested Reading

Rogers LF, Goldstein HM. Roentgen manifestations of radiation injury to the gastrointestinal tract. *Gastrointest Radiol* 1977;2:281.

Typhlitis

KEY FACTS

- Necrotizing inflammatory process that predominantly involves the cecum and right colon
- Generally occurs as a complication of leukemia, lymphoma, aplastic anemia, immunosuppressant drug therapy after organ transplantation, or AIDS
- Variable complex of fever, nausea, vomiting, and abdominal pain
- Early diagnosis and treatment with high-dose antibiotics and intravenous fluids are essential since untreated disease progresses rapidly to transmural necrosis and perforation (high mortality rate)
- On plain films, dilated atonic cecum and right colon
- On barium studies, rigidity, narrowing, and distortion of the cecum or a rigid tubular pattern with loss of haustrations involving the entire right colon
- On CT, circumferential thickening of the cecal wall (may be low-attenuation due to edema and necrosis), occasionally with intramural pneumatosis

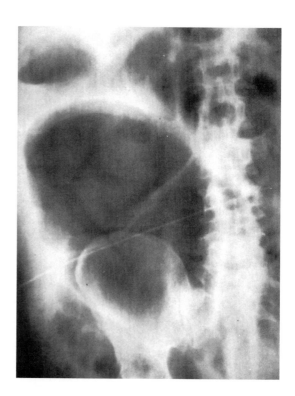

FIGURE 16-25

Typhlitis. Distended gas-filled cecum (toxic cecitis). (From Cronin TG, Calandra JD, Del Fava RL. Typhlitis presenting as toxic cecitis. *Radiology* 1981;138:29, with permission.)

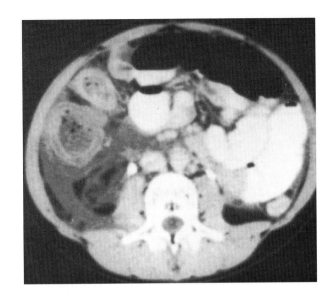

FIGURE 16-26

Typhlitis. CT scan shows that the cecal wall is thickened and contains a hypodense central layer of inflammation and edema. Note the pericecal inflammatory changes posteromedial to the cecum. (From Moss AA, Gamsu G, Genant HK, eds. *Computed tomography of the body with magnetic resonance imaging.* Philadelphia: WB Saunders, 1992, with permission.)

Suggested Reading

Cronin TG, Calandra JD, Del Fava RL. Typhlitis presenting as toxic cecitis. *Radiology* 1981; 138:29.

17 Neoplasms

Colonic Polyps

HYPERPLASTIC POLYPS

KEY FACTS

- Focal epithelial proliferation of colonic mucosa
- No malignant potential
- Smooth, sessile mucosal elevation (typically <5 mm)

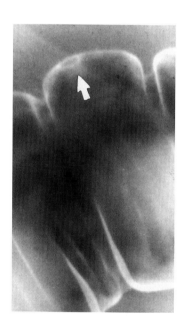

FIGURE 17-1
Hyperplastic polyp. Smooth, sessile 2-cm mucosal
elevation *(arrow)*.

Suggested Reading
Gore RM, Levine MS, Laufer I, eds. *Textbook of gastrointestinal radiology.* Philadelphia: WB
Saunders, 1994.

ADENOMATOUS POLYPS

KEY FACTS

- True neoplasm composed of branching glandular tubules lined by well-differentiated, mucus-secreting goblet cells
- Increasing incidence with advancing age
- Sessile, protuberant, or pedunculated appearance (often multiple)
- Premalignant condition:
    a. <5 mm polyp—<0.5% incidence of malignancy
    b. 5–9 mm polyp—1% incidence of malignancy
    c. 1–2 cm polyp—10% incidence of malignancy
    d. >2 cm polyp—50% incidence of malignancy
- Radiographic findings suggestive of malignancy include:
    a. irregular, lobulated surface
    b. broad base (width of base > height)
    c. retraction or indentation (puckering) of colon wall
    d. interval growth

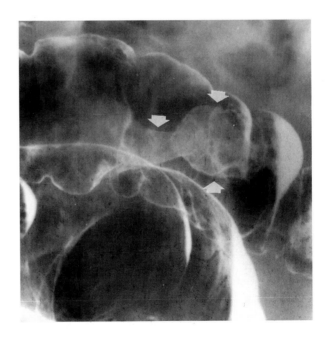

FIGURE 17-2
Adenomatous polyp.
Pedunculated mass *(arrows)*
measuring 2 cm.

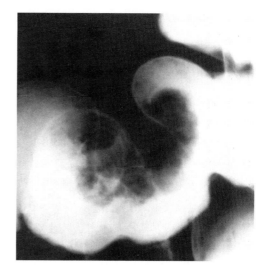

FIGURE 17-3
Malignant transformation of an
adenomatous polyp. The polyp has an
irregular, lobulated surface and there is
retraction or indentation (puckering) of the
colon wall.

Suggested Reading
Gore RM, Levine MS, Laufer I, eds. *Textbook of gastrointestinal radiology.* Philadelphia: WB
    Saunders, 1994.

HAMARTOMATOUS POLYPS

KEY FACTS

- Non-neoplastic tumor-like lesion containing abnormal quantities of normal elements
- *Peutz-Jeghers* polyp
  a. composed of branching bands of smooth muscle covered by colonic epithelium
  b. complex nodular surface that often resembles the head of a cauliflower (reflecting its arborizing infrastructure)
  c. no malignant potential

  Juvenile polyp
  a. composed of an expanded lamina propria containing mucus-filled glands but without muscularis mucosa
  b. smooth, round, usually pedunculated
  c. no malignant potential (tends to autoamputate or regress)

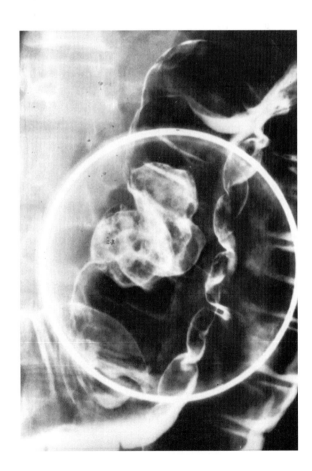

FIGURE 17-4
Hamartomatous polyp. Large lobulated mass (solitary Peutz-Jeghers polyp) in the proximal limb of the splenic flexure in a teenage boy. (From Buck JL, Harned RK, Lichtenstein JE. Peutz-Jeghers syndrome. *Radiographics* 1992; 12:365, with permission.)

Suggested Reading

Buck JL, Harned RK, Lichtenstein JE. Peutz-Jeghers syndrome. *Radiographics* 1992;12:365.

Polyposis Syndromes

KEY FACTS

- Should be suspected if:
  a. polyp is demonstrated in a young patient
  b. multiple polyps are found in any patient
  c. carcinoma of the colon occurs in a patient <40 years old

FAMILIAL POLYPOSIS

KEY FACTS

- Multiple adenomatous polyps (almost exclusively limited to the colon and rectum)
- Autosomal dominant
- 100% risk of developing colorectal cancer (40% at time of diagnosis)
- Total colectomy is usually recommended because of the high risk of malignancy

FIGURE 17-5

Familial polyposis. Innumerable adenomatous polyps blanket the entire length of the colon. The overall pattern simulates diffuse fecal material in a "poorly prepared" colon.

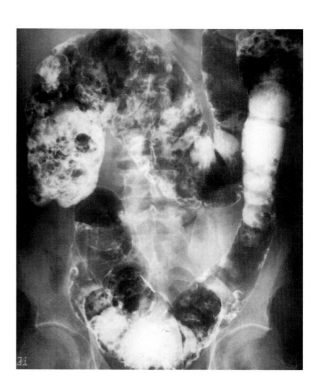

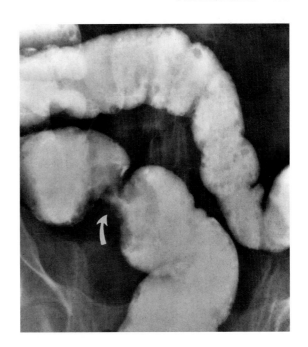

FIGURE 17-6
Sigmoid carcinoma *(arrow)*
complicating long-standing familial
polyposis.

Suggested Reading
Bartram CI, Thornton A: Colonic polyp patterns in familial polyposis. *AJR* 1984;142:305.

GARDNER'S SYNDROME

KEY FACTS

- Multiple adenomatous polyps (distribution identical to familial polyposis)
- Autosomal dominant
- 100% risk of developing colorectal cancer (total colectomy recommended)
- Associated extra-intestinal findings include:
  a. osteomas (paranasal sinuses, mandible)
  b. soft-tissue lesions (sebaceous cysts, desmoid tumors, adenomas of the upper gastrointestinal tract)
- Substantially increased risk of developing periampullary duodenal carcinoma

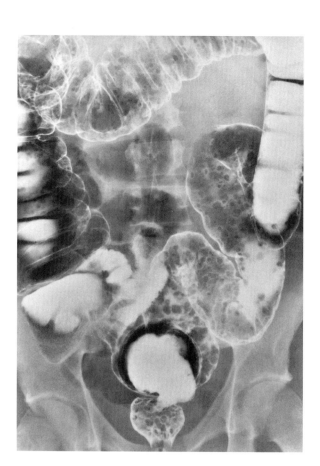

FIGURE 17-7

Gardner's syndrome. Innumerable adenomatous polyps throughout the colon present a radiographic appearance indistinguishable from familial polyposis.

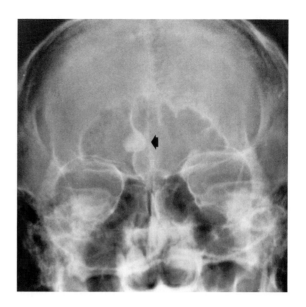

FIGURE 17-8
Gardner's syndrome. Osteoma
(arrow) in the frontal sinus.

Suggested Reading
Dolan KD, Seibert J, Seibert RW. Gardner's syndrome. *AJR* 1973;119:359.

PEUTZ-JEGHER'S SYNDROME

KEY FACTS

- Multiple hamartomatous polyps (primarily involving the small bowel)
- Most patients also have gastric and colonic polyps
- Autosomal dominant
- Polyps have no malignant potential (though 2% of patients develop gastrointestinal carcinoma elsewhere and 5% of women have ovarian cysts or tumors)
- Characteristic mucocutaneous pigmentation (especially involving the lips and buccal mucosa)

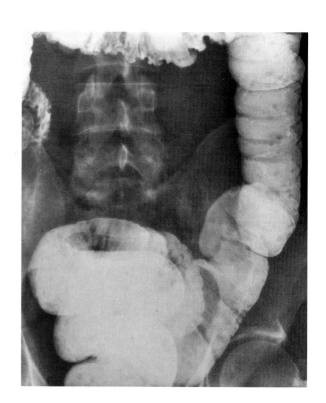

FIGURE 17-9
Peutz-Jegher's syndrome. Multiple colonic hamartomas in a patient who also demonstrated abnormal mucocutaneous pigmentation.

Suggested Reading

Buck JL, Harned RK, Lichtenstein JE, et al. Peutz-Jeghers syndrome. *Radiographics* 1992;12: 365.

CRONKHITE-CANADA SYNDROME

KEY FACTS

- Multiple nonhereditary hamartomatous juvenile polyps
- Polyps have no malignant potential
- Presents later in life with malabsorption and severe diarrhea
- Associated hyperpigmentation, alopecia, and atrophy of the fingernails and toenails
- Usually relentlessly progressive (especially in women), leading to death with 1 year of diagnosis

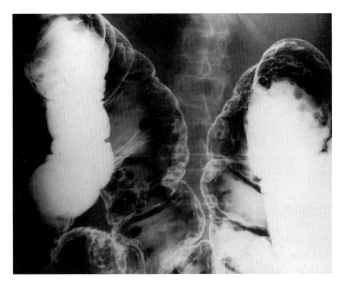

FIGURE 17-10 Cronkhite-Canada syndrome. Multiple polypoid lesions simulate familial polyposis. (From Dodds WJ. Clinical and roentgen features of the intestinal polyposis syndromes. *Gastrointest Radiol* 1976;1: 127, with permission.)

Suggested Reading

Dachman AH, Buck JL, Burke AP, et al.Cronkhite-Canada syndrome: radiologic features. *Gastrointest Radiol* 1989;14:285.

TURCOT SYNDROME

KEY FACTS

- Multiple adenomatous polyps (limited to the colon and rectum)
- Autosomal recessive
- 100% risk of developing colorectal cancer (but usually die from CNS tumor)
- Associated malignant brain tumors (usually supratentorial glioblastoma)

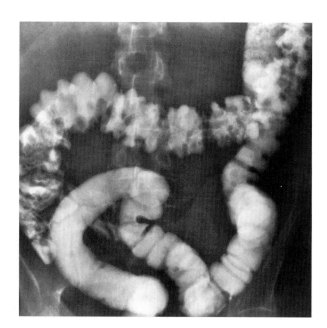

FIGURE 17-11
Turcot syndrome. Multiple adenomatous polyps in a young patient who died of malignant glioma.

Suggested Reading

Radin DR, Fortgang KC, Zee CS, et al. Turcot syndrome. A case with spinal cord and colonic neoplasms. *AJR* 1984;142:475.

MULTIPLE JUVENILE POLYPS

KEY FACTS

- Childhood disorder with no malignant potential
- Polyps tend to autoamputate or regress
- Surgery is indicated only if there are significant or repeated episodes of rectal bleeding or intussusception

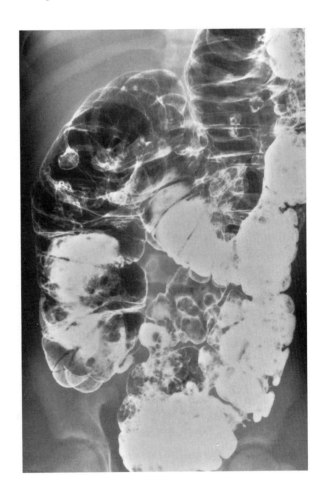

FIGURE 17-12
Multiple juvenile polyps. (From Gore RM, Levine MS, Laufer I. *Textbook of gastrointestinal radiology.* Philadelphia: WB Saunders, 1994, with permission.)

Suggested Reading

Schwartz AM, McCauley RGK. Juvenile gastrointestinal polyposis. *Radiology* 1976;121:441.

Villous Adenoma of the Colon

KEY FACTS

- Exophytic tumor consisting of innumerable villous fronds that give the surface a corrugated appearance
- Typically solitary and located in the rectosigmoid area
- About 40% demonstrate infiltrating carcinoma (usually at the base)
- Bulky tumor with virtually pathognomonic appearance of barium filling the interstices of the mass (between the multiple fronds)
- Profound mucous diarrhea may cause severe fluid, protein, and electrolyte depletion

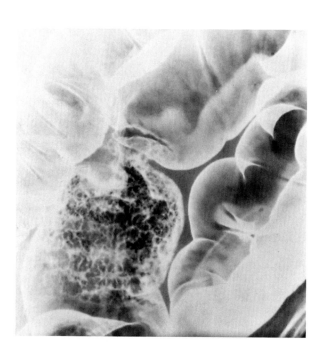

FIGURE 17-13

Villous adenoma. Fine lace-like pattern resulting from seepage of barium into interstices between individual tumor fronds. The bulk of the rectal tumor expands the lumen; a notch on the right superolateral aspect represents the point of attachment. (From Margulis AR, Burhenne HJ, eds. *Alimentary tract radiology.* St. Louis: Mosby, 1983, with permission.)

Suggested Reading

Delamarre J, Descombes P, Marti R, et al. Villous tumors of the colon and rectum: double-contrast study of 47 cases. *Gastrointest Radiol* 1980;5:69.

Lipoma of the Colon

KEY FACTS

- Most common benign submucosal colonic tumor
- Frequently presents as the lead point of an intussusception
- Smooth submucosal filling defect that is usually single and most often involves the right colon
- Fatty consistency makes the tumor changeable in size and shape with palpation

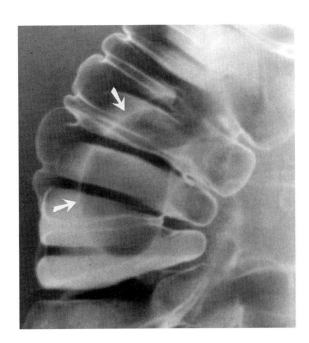

FIGURE 17-14

Lipoma. Extremely lucent mass with smooth margins and a teardrop shape *(arrows)*.

Suggested Reading

Taylor AJ, Stewart ET, Dodds WJ. Gastrointestinal lipomas: a radiologic and pathologic review. *AJR* 1990;155:1205.

Carcinoma of the Colon

KEY FACTS

- Most common cancer of the gastrointestinal tract and second most common cause of death from malignancy (after lung cancer in men and breast cancer in women)
- Overall 5-year survival rate of 40% to 50%
- Risk factors include:
  a. adenomatous/villous colonic polyps
  b. familial polyposis/Gardner's syndrome
  c. chronic ulcerative colitis
  d. refined, low-fiber diet
- Radiographic findings include:
  a. annular constricting lesion with ulcerated mucosa, eccentric and irregular lumen, and overhanging margins ("apple core")
  b. flat plaque of tumor involving only a portion of the circumference of the colon wall ("saddle" lesion)
  c. discrete intraluminal polyp
  d. fungating polypoid mass
  e. scirrhous (long circumferential narrowing often seen as a complication of chronic ulcerative colitis)
- 1% risk of multiple synchronous colon cancers; 3% risk of metachronous cancers
- CT is the imaging modality of choice for staging colon carcinoma and assessing tumor recurrence

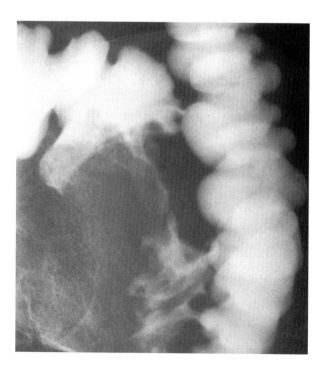

FIGURE 17-15

Carcinoma of the colon. Annular constricting lesion with overhanging margins.

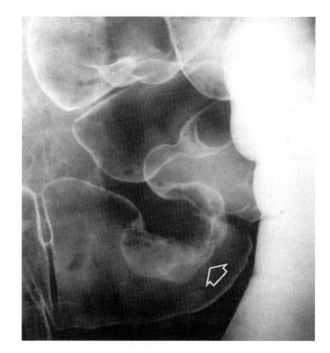

FIGURE 17-16
Carcinoma of the colon (saddle cancer). The tumor *(arrow)* appears to sit on the upper margin of the distal transverse colon like a saddle on a horse.

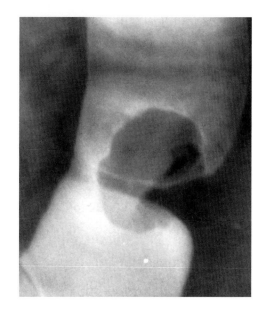

FIGURE 17-17
Carcinoma of the colon. Large sessile mass with an irregular lobulated surface.

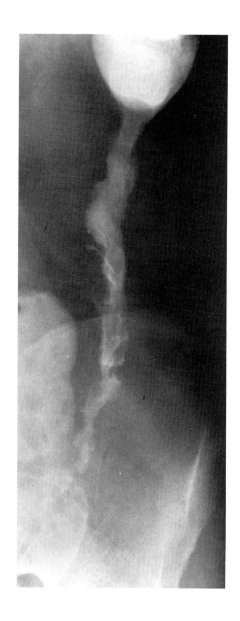

FIGURE 17-18

Scirrhous cancer of the colon. Severe
circumferential narrowing of a long segment of
the descending colon.

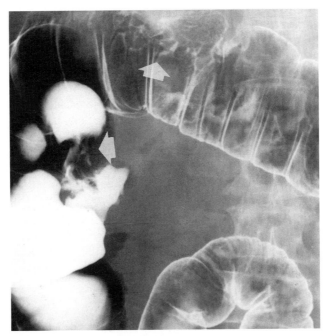

A

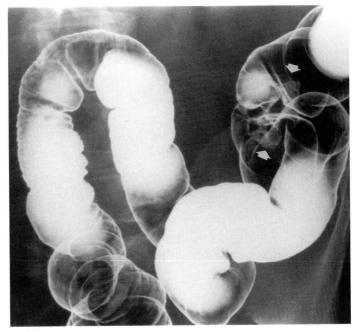

B

FIGURE 17-19   Multiple synchronous carcinomas of the colon. **A:** Carcinomas of the ascending and transverse portions of the colon *(arrows)*.
B: Carcinoma *(arrows)* within a tortuous descending colon.

Suggested Reading

Gore RM, Levine MS, Laufer I, eds. *Textbook of gastrointestinal radiology.* Philadelphia: WB Saunders, 1994.

Metastases to the Colon

KEY FACTS

- Major sources include:
  a. direct invasion (prostate, ovary, uterus, cervix, kidney, gallbladder)
  b. via mesenteric reflections (stomach, pancreas)
  c. intraperitoneal seeding (especially involving the pouch of Douglas, inferomedial border of the cecum, right paracolic gutter, and sigmoid mesocolon)
  d. hematogenous spread (melanoma, carcinomas of the breast and lung)
  e. lymphangitic spread (infrequent)
- Various radiographic patterns including marginal and deep ulcerations, nodular extrinsic masses, annular or eccentric strictures, long infiltrative segments of irregular narrowing, and the "striped colon" (transverse folds that do not completely traverse the colonic lumen)

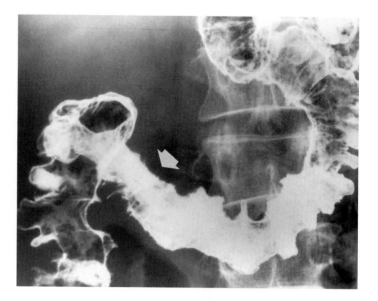

FIGURE 17-20   Metastases to the colon (gastric carcinoma). Irregular narrowing and spiculation involve the proximal transverse colon.

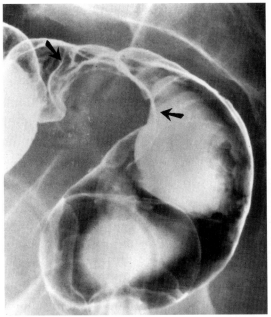

A

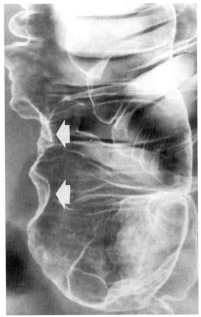

B

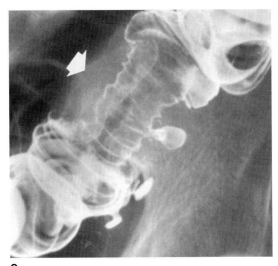

C

FIGURE 17-21
Intraperitoneal metastatic seeding
involving the colon *(arrows)*.
A: Pouch of Douglas. **B:** Lateral
aspect of the cecum in the right
paracolic gutter. **C:** Superior border of
the sigmoid colon.

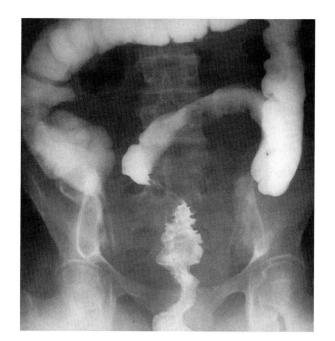

FIGURE 17-22

Metastases to the colon (ovarian cystadenocarcinoma). Mass effect combined with a desmoplastic reaction that causes tethering of mucosal folds and an annular stricture.

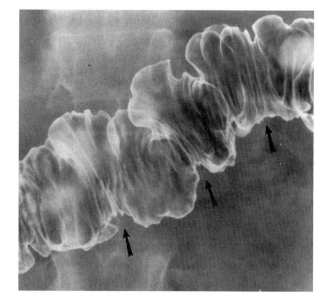

FIGURE 17-23

Metastases to the colon (striped colon sign). Numerous transverse folds of the transverse colon *(arrows)*. (From Ginaldi S, Lindell MM, Zornoza J. The striped colon: a new radiographic observation in metastatic serosal implants. *AJR* 1980;134:453, with permission.)

Suggested Reading

Rubesin SE, Levine MS. Omental cakes: colonic involvement by omental metastases. *Radiology* 1985;154:593.

18 Other Disorders

Toxic Megacolon

KEY FACTS

- Dramatic and ominous complication of acute fulminant ulcerating disease of the colon
- Most frequently develops during relapses of chronic ulcerative colitis
- Characterized by extreme dilatation (>6 cm) of a segment of colon (usually the transverse) combined with systemic toxicity
- Multiple broad-based nodular pseudopolypoid projections are often seen extending into the lumen
- Barium enema is contraindicated
- On CT, the wall of the distended colon is thin but has a nodular contour; intramural gas may occur
- Spontaneous perforation of the colon occurs in up to 50% of cases; mortality rate of 20% to 30%

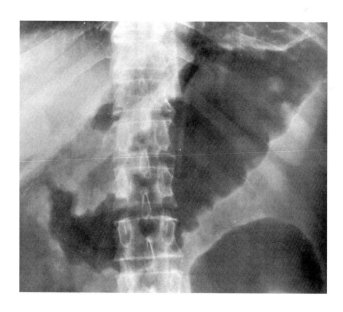

FIGURE 18-1
Toxic megacolon. Dilatation of the transverse colon with multiple pseudopolypoid projections extending into the lumen.

Suggested Reading
Halpert RD. Toxic dilatation of the colon. *Radiol Clin North Am* 1987;25:147.

Diverticulosis

KEY FACTS

- Acquired herniations of mucosa and submucosa through the muscular layers of the bowel wall
- Incidence increases with age (rare <30; up to 50% in those >60)
- Primarily involves the sigmoid colon
- Diverticula usually develop between the mesenteric and lateral taenia at sites of weakness in the colon wall, where the longitudinal arteries penetrate the inner circular muscle layer to form the submucosal capillary plexus
- Generally asymptomatic, but may cause painless rectal bleeding (may be brisk and life-threatening)
- Multiple round or oval outpouchings of barium projecting beyond the lumen
- Criss-crossing ridges of thickened circular muscle can produce a series of sacculations (sawtooth configuration)
- On CT, muscle hypertrophy appears as a thickened colon wall with distorted luminal contours; diverticula are seen as well-defined gas- or contrast-filled sacs outside the colon lumen

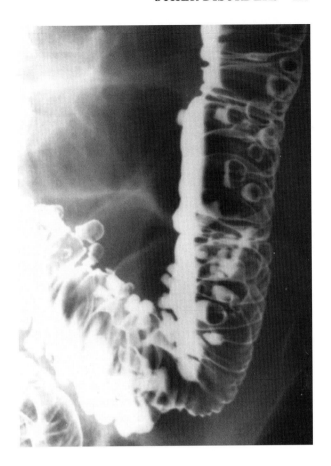

FIGURE 18-2
Diverticulosis. Multiple barium-coated, air-filled diverticula superimposed on the bowel lumen mimic discrete colonic filling defects.

Suggested Reading
Almy TP, Howell DA. Diverticular disease of the colon. *N Engl J Med* 1980;302:324.

Diverticulitis

KEY FACTS

- Complication of diverticulosis in which a micro- or macroperforation of a diverticulum leads to the development of a peridiverticular abscess
- Typically involves the sigmoid region and produces left lower quadrant pain and tenderness, a palpable mass, fever, and leukocytosis
- Definitive radiographic diagnosis requires evidence of diverticular perforation:
  - a. extravasation of contrast material
    or
  - b. eccentric narrowing (by a pericolic mass due to a localized abscess representing a walled-off perforation)
- Other radiographic findings include "double tracking" (sinus tract extending along the colon) and fistulas to the bladder, small bowel, or vagina
- May be indistinguishable from carcinoma (though in diverticulitis the area of narrowing is usually longer with intact, though often distorted, mucosa and tapering margins)
- CT findings include:
  - a. circumferential thickening of the bowel wall
  - b. inflammation of pericolic fat
  - c. peridiverticular abscess
  - d. intramural sinus tracts
  - e. induration and thickening of the sigmoid mesocolon

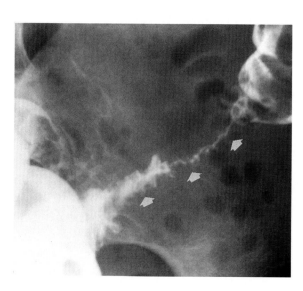

FIGURE 18-3

Diverticulitis. Severe spasm and adjacent walled-off abscess cause marked narrowing of the colonic lumen *(arrows).*

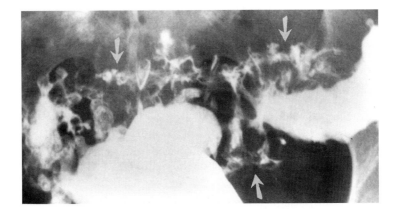

FIGURE 18-4   Diverticulitis. Extraluminal tracks extend along both the mesocolic *(upper arrows)* and antimesocolic *(lower arrow)* borders of the sigmoid colon.

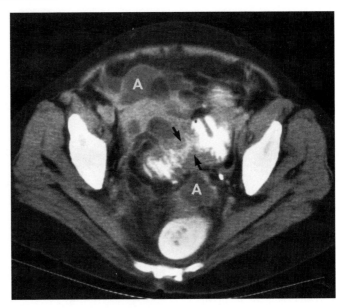

FIGURE 18-5   Diverticulitis. CT scan shows narrowing of the lumen of the sigmoid colon *(arrows)* and multiple adjacent pericolonic abscesses *(A)*.

Suggested Reading

Cho KC, Morehouse HT, Alterman DD, et al. Sigmoid diverticulitis: diagnostic role of CT— comparison with barium enema studies. *Radiology* 1990;176:111.

Volvulus of the Colon

CECAL VOLVULUS

KEY FACTS

- Twist of the cecum on its axis that develops in some patients with a long mesentery (hypermobile cecum)
- Distended cecum is displaced upward and to the left, appearing as a kidney-shaped mass with the torqued and thickened mesentery mimicking the renal pelvis
- Barium enema demonstrates obstruction of the contrast column at the level of the stenosis, with the tapered edge of the column pointing toward the site of torsion

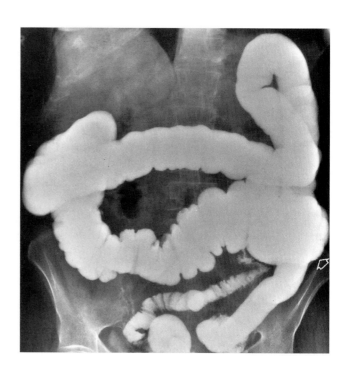

FIGURE 18-6
Hypermobile cecum. The unusually long mesentery permits the cecum and ascending colon to course horizontally, with the tip of the cecum *(arrow)* near the left wall of the abdomen.

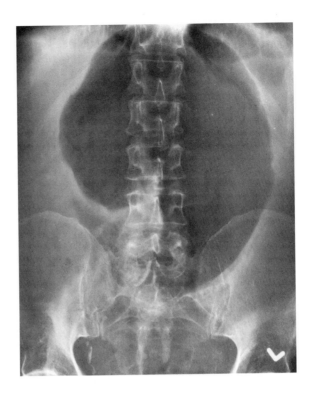

FIGURE 18-7
Cecal volvulus. The distended, gas-
filled cecum is displaced upward
and to the left.

Suggested Reading
Kerry RL, Lee F, Ransom HK: Roentgenologic examination in the diagnosis and treatment of
colon volvulus. *AJR* 1971;113:343.

SIGMOID VOLVULUS

KEY FACTS

- Twist of a long, redundant loop of sigmoid colon on its mesenteric axis, resulting in a closed-loop obstruction
- Inverted U-shaped shadow that rises out of the pelvis in a vertical or oblique direction
- Barium enema demonstrates obstruction of the contrast column, with the lumen tapering toward the site of stenosis ("bird's beak" appearance)
- Rectal tube decompression is the preferred form of initial treatment if there are no signs of vascular compromise
- High recurrence rate (up to 80%) often requires surgical resection of the redundant sigmoid

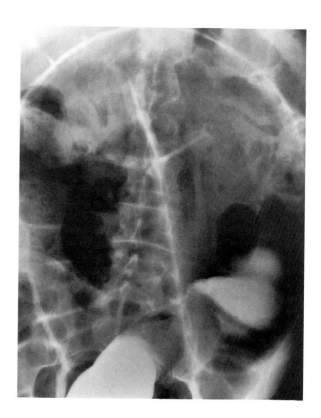

FIGURE 18-8

Sigmoid volvulus. Massively dilated loop of sigmoid appears as an inverted U-shaped shadow rising out of the pelvis.

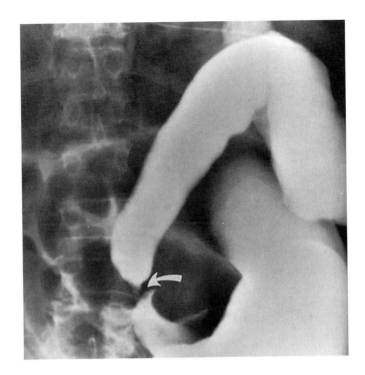

FIGURE 18-9   Sigmoid volvulus. Barium enema demonstrates luminal tapering at the site of stenosis, producing a characteristic "bird's-beak" configuration.

Suggested Reading
Love L. Large bowel obstruction. *Semin Roentgenol* 1973;8:299.

Aganglionosis of the Colon (Hirschsprung's Disease)

KEY FACTS

- Absence of parasympathetic ganglia in muscular and submucosal layers
- Typically involves a short segment of rectosigmoid
- Massive dilatation of the colon with prolonged retention of fecal material proximally
- Rectum usually of normal caliber (though it is the abnormal segment) and an abrupt transition to the area of grossly dilated bowel (which has normal innervation)

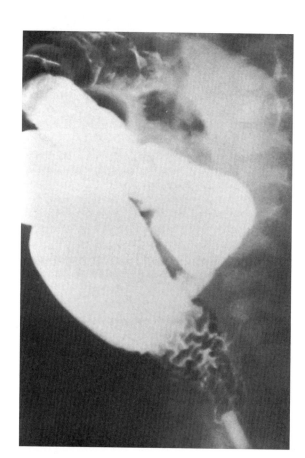

FIGURE 18-10

Aganglionosis (Hirschsprung's disease). Lateral view from a barium enema shows a corrugated appearance of the rectum with huge dilatation of the sigmoid colon. (From Gore RM, Levine MS, Laufer I. *Textbook of gastrointestinal radiology.* Philadelphia: WB Saunders, 1994, with permission.)

Suggested Reading

Rosenfield NS, Ablow RC, Markowitz RK, et al. Hirschsprung's disease: accuracy of the barium enema examination. *Radiology* 1984;150:393.

Colitis Cystica Profunda

KEY FACTS

- Large submucosal mucus-containing cysts lined by normal colonic mucosa
- Typically involves a short segment of sigmoid or rectum
- Benign condition with no malignant potential
- Multiple irregular filling defects (single mass may mimic sessile polyp)
- Barium-filled clefts between nodules produces spiculations mimicking ulcers

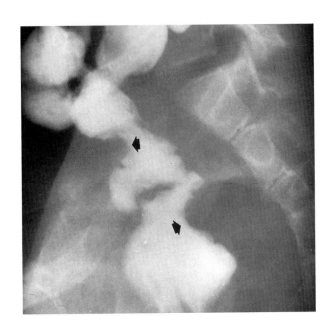

FIGURE 18-11
Colitis cystica profunda. Multiple submucosal filling defects *(arrows)* in the rectum associated with widening of the retrorectal space. (From Ledesma-Medina J, Reid BS, Girdany BR. Colitis cystica profunda. *AJR* 1978;131:529, with permission.)

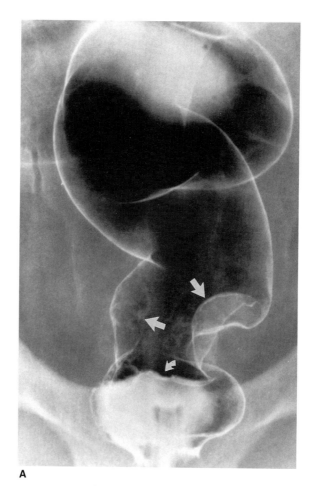

A

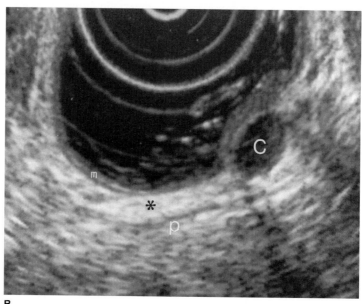

B

FIGURE 18-12 Colitis cystica profunda. **A:** Three well-demarcated cystic submucosal lesions *(arrows)* protruding into the rectal lumen. The distal lesion, just above the anal verge on the posterior wall, shows an irregularly ulcerated contour radiographically suggestive of carcinoma. **B:** Transrectal ultrasound of one of the lesions shows mucosa covering a mucus-filled cyst (C), located mainly in the submucosa. There is no disruption of the deeper layers. *M*, mucosa; *p*, muscularis propria; *asterisk*, submucosa. (From Hulsmans FJH, Tio TL, Reeders JWAJ, et al. Transrectal US in the diagnosis of localized colitis cystica profunda. *Radiology* 1991;181:201, with permission.)

Suggested Reading

Hulsman FJH, Tio TL, Reeders JWAJ, et al. Transrectal US in the diagnosis of localized colitis cystica profunda. *Radiology* 1991;181:201.

Pelvic Lipomatosis

KEY FACTS

- Benign increased deposition of normal mature adipose tissue with minimal fibrotic/inflammatory components that compresses soft-tissue structures within the pelvis
- Strong male predominance and not related to obesity
- Major complication is ureteral obstruction (40% within 5 years)
- Increased pelvic lucency on plain radiographs (confirmed on CT)
- Vertical elongation of the sigmoid colon with narrowing of the rectum and sigmoid by the extrinsic fatty mass
- Characteristic teardrop- or pear-shaped bladder

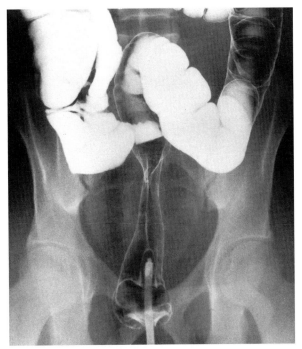

A

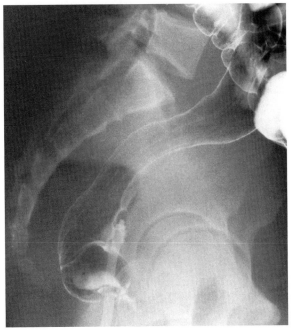

FIGURE 18-13
Pelvic lipomatosis. Frontal (**A**)
and lateral (**B**) views show
smooth narrowing of the rectum
and proximal sigmoid colon.

B

Suggested Reading
Crane DB, Smith MJV. Pelvic lipomatosis: five-year follow-up. *J Urol* 1977;118:547.

GALLBLADDER AND BILIARY TREE

19   Gallbladder

Gallstones (Cholelithiasis)

KEY FACTS

- Can develop whenever bile contains insufficient bile salts and lecithin in proportion to cholesterol to maintain the cholesterol in solution
- Approximately 80% are lucent cholesterol stones; 20% contain sufficient calcium to be radiographically detectable
- Increased incidence in women and patients with hemolytic anemias, cirrhosis, diabetes, Crohn's disease, hyperparathyroidism, or pancreatitis
- Freely movable and settle in the dependent portion of the gallbladder (level depends on the relationship between the specific gravity of the stone to that of the surrounding bile)
- On ultrasound, a high-amplitude intraluminal echo associated with posterior acoustic shadowing
- A gallbladder completely filled with stones with no lumen identified (about 20% of cases) may be diagnosed by demonstrating a high-amplitude echo associated with a posterior acoustic shadow
- Bile sludge appears as a nonshadowing, echogenic, homogeneous viscous mass that moves slowly with changes in the patient's position

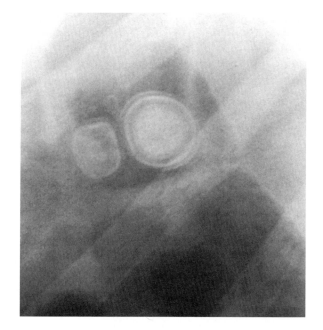

FIGURE 19-1

Laminated gallstones. Alternating lucent and opaque layers. (From Gedgaudas-McClees RK, ed. *Handbook of gastrointestinal imaging.* New York: Churchill Livingstone, 1987, with permission.)

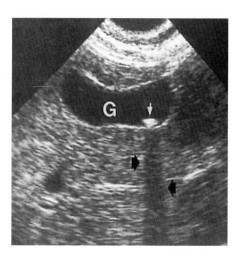

FIGURE 19-2

Gallstones. The anechoic gallbladder *(G)* contains an echogenic focus, representing a large gallstone *(white arrow)*. Note the acoustic shadowing immediately inferior to the stone *(black arrows)*.

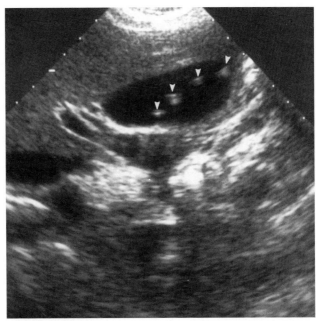

A

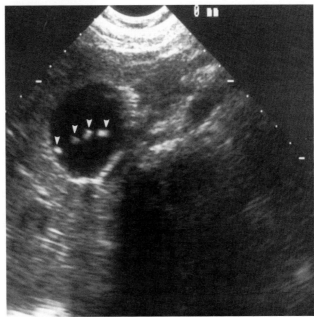

B

FIGURE 19-3

Floating gallstones. Sagittal **(A)** and transverse **(B)** scans show multiple hyperechoic structures *(arrowheads)* floating in the lumen of the gallbladder. (From Krebs CA, Giyanani VL, Eisenberg RL. *Ultrasound atlas of disease processes.* Norwalk, CT: Appleton & Lange, 1993, with permission.)

F I G U R E 1 9 - 4

Gallstones with nonvisualization of the gallbladder lumen. Hyperechoic structure in the gallbladder fossa *(arrow)* with acoustic shadowing, though the gallbladder lumen is not visualized. (From Krebs CA, Giyanani VL, Eisenberg RL. *Ultrasound atlas of disease processes.* Norwalk, CT: Appleton & Lange, 1993, with permission.)

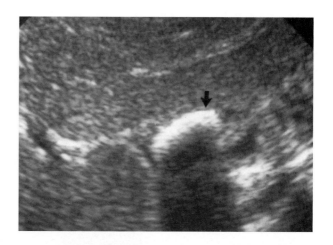

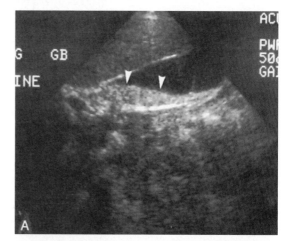

F I G U R E 1 9 - 5

Sludge. The homogeneous hypoechoic material *(arrowheads)* moves as the patient moves from the supine **(A)** to the decubitus **(B)** position. Note the absence of distal shadowing. (From Cohen SM, Kurtz AB. Biliary sonography. *Radiol Clin North Am* 1991;29:1171, with permission.)

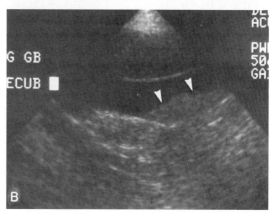

Suggested Reading

Cohen SM, Kurtz AB. Biliary sonography. *Radiol Clin North Am* 1991;29:1171.

Cholecystitis

ACUTE CHOLECYSTITIS

KEY FACTS

- In about 90%, related to cystic duct obstruction by an impacted calculus
- On ultrasound, thickening of the gallbladder wall (>3 mm) is usually associated with a densely echogenic stone, posterior acoustic shadowing, and pericholecystic fluid
- Three-layered wall thickening, with a hypoechoic region (subserosal edema and necrosis) sandwiched between two echogenic lines (may also be a striated pattern)
- Thickened gallbladder wall is not specific and can also be seen in such conditions as incomplete fasting, hypoalbuminemia, ascites, and congestive heart failure
- Sonographic Murphy's sign (pain on compression of the gallbladder with the ultrasound transducer)
- On radionuclide scanning, prompt tracer accumulation in the liver and excretion into the bowel, but no visualization of the gallbladder at 4 hours

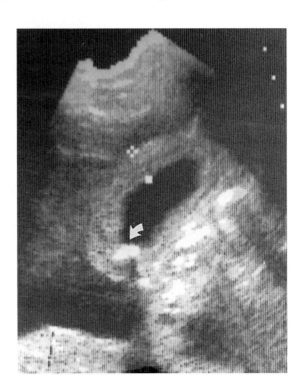

FIGURE 19-6
Acute cholecystitis. Marked thickening of the gallbladder wall (1.1 cm between the cursors). There is a densely echogenic stone *(arrow)* with posterior acoustic shadowing in the neck of the gallbladder.

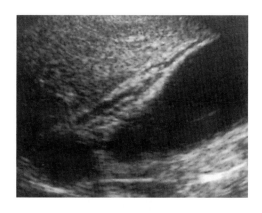

FIGURE 19-7

Acute gangrenous cholecystitis. Striated (layered) thickening of the gallbladder wall, in which multiple hypoechoic layers *(arrowheads)* are separated by echogenic zones. [From Teefey SA, Baron RL, Bigler SA. Sonography of the gallbladder: significance of striated (layered) thickening of the gallbladder wall. *AJR* 1991;156:945, with permission.]

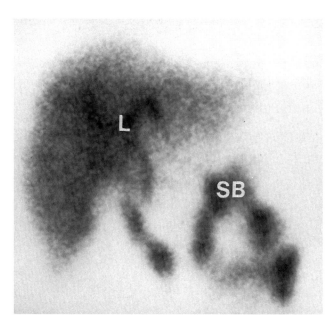

FIGURE 19-8

Acute cholecystitis. On this delayed film from a radionuclide hepatobiliary scan, there is normal activity and excretion through the liver *(L)* and small bowel *(SB)* but persistent nonvisualization of the gallbladder. (From Krebs CA, Giyanani VL, Eisenberg RL. *Ultrasound atlas of disease processes.* Norwalk, CT: Appleton & Lange, 1993, with permission.)

Suggested Reading

Teefey SA, Baron RL, Bigler SA. Sonography of the gallbladder: significance of striated (layered) thickening of the gallbladder wall. *AJR* 1991;156:945.

ACALCULOUS CHOLECYSTITIS

KEY FACTS

- Those 10% of cases of acute cholecystitis in which no gallstone can be identified
- Probably related to decreased blood supply through the cystic artery secondary to:
  a. depressed motility or starvation (trauma, burns, surgery, total parenteral nutrition, narcotics, shock)
  b. extrinsic inflammation of the cystic duct (inflammation, lymphadenopathy, metastases)
  c. infection
- Patients at risk include those with biliary stasis due to lack of oral intake or total parenteral nutrition, or following trauma or surgery
- On ultrasound, distended and tender gallbladder with a thickened wall but without stones
- On radionuclide scanning, lack of gallbladder visualization (nonspecific, since it may merely reflect total parenteral nutrition or prolonged severe illness)

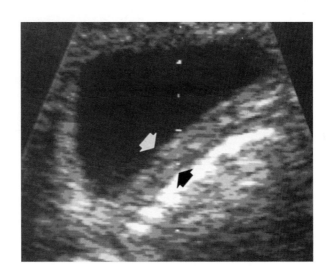

FIGURE 19-9
Acalculous cholecystitis. Enlarged gallbladder with a thickened, edematous wall *(arrows)*. There is no evidence of gallstones or posterior acoustic shadowing.

Suggested Reading
Cohen SM, Kurtz AB. Biliary sonography. *Radiol Clin North Am* 1991;29:1171.

CHRONIC CHOLECYSTITIS

KEY FACTS

- Chronic inflammation of the gallbladder with stones
- Recurrent attacks of right upper quadrant pain and biliary colic
- On ultrasound, gallstones, thickening of the gallbladder wall, contraction of the lumen, and poor contractility
- On radionuclide scanning, delayed visualization of the gallbladder

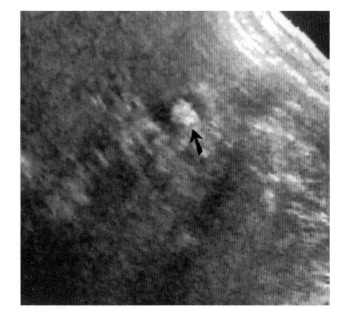

FIGURE 19-10
Chronic cholecystitis. Small contracted intrahepatic gallbladder containing a hyperechoic structure representing a gallstone *(arrow)*. (From Krebs CA, Giyanani VL, Eisenberg RL. *Ultrasound atlas of disease processes.* Norwalk, CT: Appleton & Lange, 1993, with permission.)

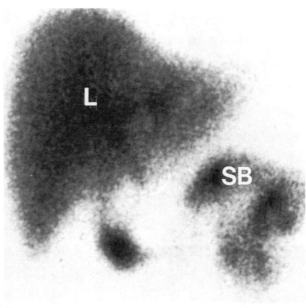

FIGURE 19-11
Chronic cholecystitis. **A:** Early radionuclide hepatobiliary scan shows nonvisualization of the gallbladder. **B:** Delayed scan shows visualization of the gallbladder *(GB)*. *L*, liver; *SB*, small bowel; *C*, colon. (From Krebs CA, Giyanani VL, Eisenberg RL. *Ultrasound atlas of disease processes.* Norwalk, CT: Appleton & Lange, 1993, with permission.)

Suggested Reading
Cohen SM, Kurtz AB. Biliary sonography. *Radiol Clin North Am* 1991;29:1171.

EMPHYSEMATOUS CHOLECYSTITIS

KEY FACTS

- Infection of the gallbladder by gas-forming organisms (*Escherichia coli, Clostridium perfringens*)
- Bacterial growth is usually facilitated by cystic duct obstruction, which causes stasis and ischemia in the gallbladder
- Up to 50% of cases occur in poorly controlled diabetics
- Collections of gas in the gallbladder lumen, wall of the gallbladder, or pericholecystic tissues
- On ultrasound, high-level echoes of gas outline the gallbladder wall, while intraluminal gas appears as an echogenic focus with ring-down artifact

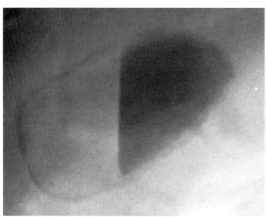

A

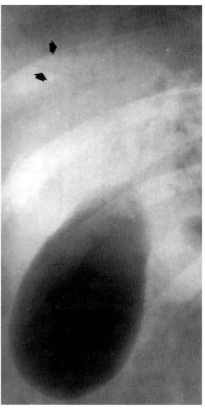

B

FIGURE 19-12

Emphysematous cholecystitis. **A:** Gas in both the lumen and wall of the gallbladder. **B:** In addition to gas filling the gallbladder lumen, there is also faintly seen gas in the portal veins *(arrows)*.

Suggested Reading

Rice RP, Thompson WM, Gedgaudas RK. The diagnosis and significance of extraluminal gas in the abdomen. *Radiol Clin North Am* 1982;20:819.

Milk of Calcium Bile

KEY FACTS

- Filling of the gallbladder with an accumulation of bile that appears opaque because of a high concentration of calcium compounds
- Secondary to chronic cholecystitis with a thickened gallbladder wall and an obstructed cystic duct
- Diffuse opacification of the gallbladder lumen (simulates a normal gallbladder filled with contrast material)
- On ultrasound, extremely echogenic bile within which gallstones may be visualized

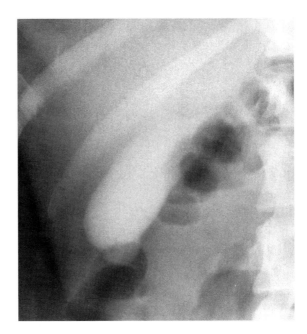

FIGURE 19-13
Milk of calcium bile. Plain abdominal radiograph demonstrates a completely opaque gallbladder in a patient who had not received any cholecystographic agent.

Suggested Reading

Eisenberg RL. *Gastrointestinal radiology: a pattern approach.* Philadelphia: Lippincott–Raven Publishers, 1996.

Porcelain Gallbladder

KEY FACTS

- Extensive mural calcification around the perimeter of the gallbladder
- Thickening and fibrosis of the underlying gallbladder wall secondary to chronic cholecystitis
- About 10% to 20% incidence of gallbladder carcinoma (therefore a prophylactic cholecystectomy is usually performed even if the patient is asymptomatic)
- On ultrasound, highly echogenic curvilinear structure with posterior shadowing in the gallbladder fossa (representing the stone-filled, contracted gallbladder)

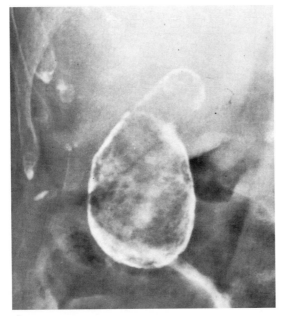

A

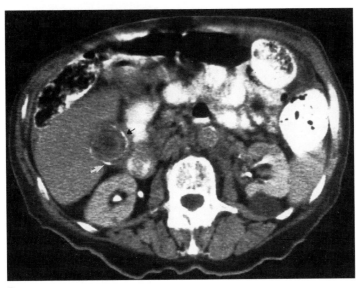

B

FIGURE 19-14   Porcelain gallbladder. **A:** Plain radiograph demonstrates extensive mural calcification around the perimeter of the gallbladder. **B:** CT scan in another patient shows calcification of the gallbladder wall *(arrows).*

Suggested Reading

Oschner SF, Carrera GM. Calcification of the gallbladder ("porcelain gallbladder"). *AJR* 1963;89:847.

Carcinoma of the Gallbladder

KEY FACTS

- Primarily affects women of age >50
- 80% to 90% have cholelithiasis
- Initially asymptomatic; when symptoms occur they usually are secondary to coexisting cholecystitis or cholelithiasis
- Rapidly progressive and invariably fatal (1-year survival <10%)
- Ultrasound and CT show a mass in the gallbladder fossa with extension to the liver
- Other imaging findings may include thickening of the gallbladder wall, a fixed intraluminal gallbladder mass, gallstones, biliary obstruction, nodal involvement, and hematogenous metastases

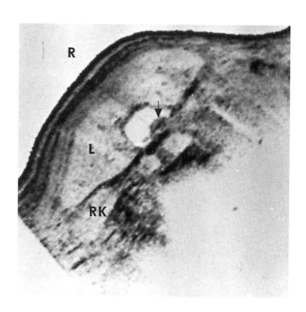

FIGURE 19-15

Carcinoma of the gallbladder. Transverse sonogram of the right upper abdomen demonstrates a focal gallbladder mass *(arrow)* that was not dependent or associated with acoustic shadowing. *RK,* right kidney. (Courtesy of Dr. James Waskey.) (From Margulis AR, Burhenne HG, eds. *Alimentary tract radiology.* St. Louis: CV Mosby, 1983, with permission.)

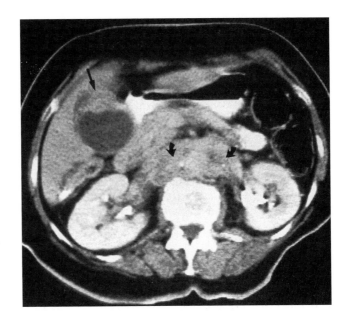

FIGURE 19-16
Carcinoma of the gallbladder.
CT scan demonstrates a soft-
tissue mass along the anterior
wall of the gallbladder
(straight arrow). Note the
paraaortic nodal metastases
(curved arrows).

Suggested Reading

Cohen SM, Kurtz AB. Biliary sonography. *Radiol Clin North Am* 1991;29:1171.

Hyperplastic Cholesteroloses

KEY FACTS

- Noninflammatory disorders consisting of benign proliferation of normal tissue elements in the gallbladder wall
- Functional abnormalities of the gallbladder include hyperconcentration, hypercontraction, and hyperexcretion
- Associated with gallstones in up to 75% of cases
- No malignant potential

CHOLESTEROLOSIS (STRAWBERRY GALLBLADDER)

KEY FACTS

- Abnormal deposits of cholesterol esters in fat-laden macrophages in the lamina propria of the gallbladder wall
- Fatty material causes coarse, yellow, speckled masses on the surface of a reddened, hyperemic gallbladder mucosa (like strawberry seeds)
- Single or multiple small polypoid filling defects in an opacified gallbladder
- On ultrasound, nonshadowing, single or multiple fixed echoes that project into the lumen of the gallbladder

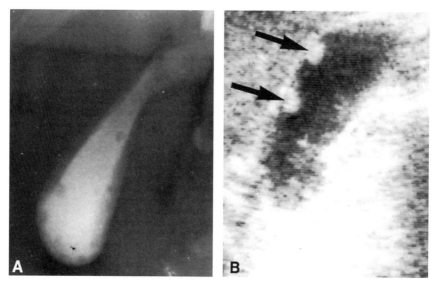

FIGURE 19-17   Cholesterolosis. Oral cholecystogram (A) and ultrasound (B) show multiple discrete small polypoid defects adherent to the gallbladder wall. There was no movement with change in position in either study. No shadowing is seen on ultrasound. (From Simeone JF. The gallbladder: pathology. In: Taveras JM, Ferrucci JT, eds. *Radiology: diagnosis—imaging intervention.* Philadelphia: JB Lippincott, 1987, with permission.)

Suggested Reading

Berk RN, van der Vegt JH, Lichtenstein JE. The hyperplastic cholecystoses: cholesterolosis and adenomyomatosis. *Radiology* 1983;146:593.

ADENOMYOMATOSIS

KEY FACTS

- Intramural diverticulosis in which there are mucosal outpouchings (Rokitansky-Aschoff sinuses) into or through a thickened muscle layer
- In the generalized form, the sinuses appear as multiple oval collections of contrast extending just outside the lumen of the gallbladder (string of beads)
- In the segmental form, a thin septum produces compartmentalization of the gallbladder
- An adenomyoma is a localized form in which there is a single, sessile, smooth filling defect situated at the tip of the fundus
- On ultrasound, focal or diffuse thickening of the gallbladder wall in association with anechoic cystic spaces (may be intraluminal septations or projections)

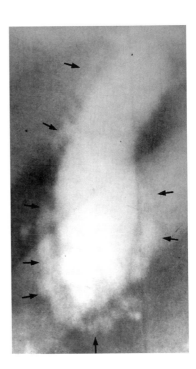

FIGURE 19-18

Adenomyomatosis. Rokitansky-Aschoff sinuses *(arrows)* are scattered diffusely throughout the gallbladder.

FIGURE 19-19

Segmental adenomyomatosis.
Localized circumferential thickening
(arrow) of the gallbladder wall.
(From Harned RL, Williams FM,
Anderson JC. Gallbladder disease.
In: Eisenberg RL, ed. *Diagnostic
imaging: an algorithmic approach.*
Philadelphia: JB Lippincott, 1988,
with permission.)

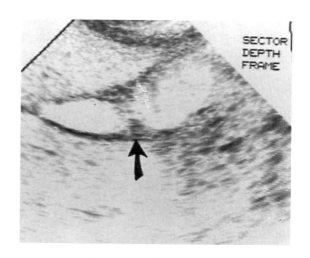

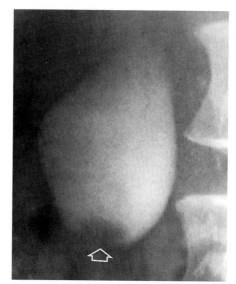

FIGURE 19-20

Solitary adenomyoma. Broad mass *(arrow)* at
the tip of the fundus of the gallbladder.

FIGURE 19-21

Adenomyomatosis. Long-
axis **(A)** and transverse **(B)**
images show wall thickening
and multiple hyperechoic
foci representing "ring
down" artifacts *(arrowheads)*
that represent Rokitansky-
Aschoff sinuses. Note the
classic shadowing gallstone
in the fundus. (From Cohen
SM, Kurtz AB. Biliary
sonography. *Radiol Clin
North Am* 1991;29:1171,
with permission.)

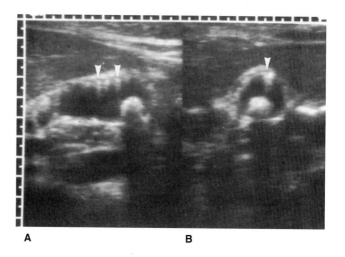

A   B

Suggested Reading

Jutras JA, Levesque HP. Adenomyoma and adenomyomatosis of the gallbladder: radiologic
and pathologic correlations. *Radiol Clin North Am* 1966;4:483.

20   Bile Ducts

Choledocholithiasis

KEY FACTS

- Usually arises in the gallbladder and reaches the bile duct either by passage through the cystic duct or by fistulous erosion through the gallbladder wall
- Single or multiple filling defects in the opacified biliary tree that move freely and change location with alterations in patient position
- May impact in the distal common duct and cause obstruction (smooth, sharply defined meniscus)
- Ultrasound can image about 90% of proximal duct and 70% of distal duct stones
- Most common duct stones are echogenic structures that cast an acoustic shadow (about 10% do not shadow)
- CT demonstrates characteristic target and crescent signs

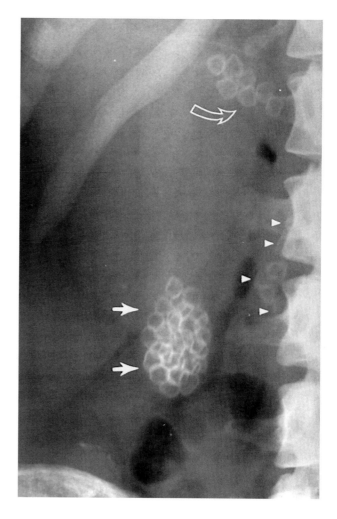

FIGURE 20-1
Choledocholithiasis. Multiple calculi in the common bile duct *(open arrow)*, some of which overlie the spine and are difficult to detect *(arrowheads)*. Note the associated calculi in the gallbladder *(solid arrows)*. (From Baker SR, Elkin M. *Plain film approach to abdominal calcifications.* Philadelphia: WB Saunders, 1983, with permission.)

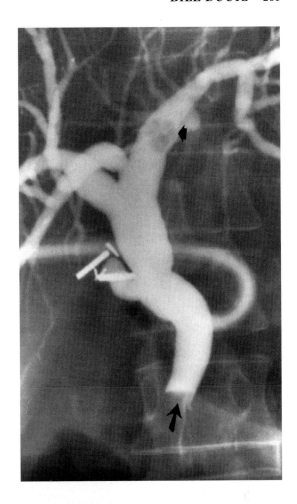

FIGURE 20-2

Impacted ampullary stone. Smooth, sharply defined meniscus in the distal common bile duct *(long arrow)*. Note the second stone *(short arrow)* in the left hepatic duct.

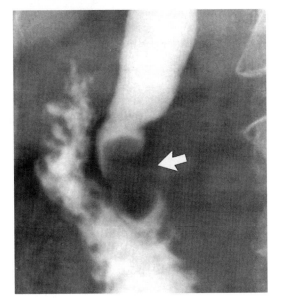

FIGURE 20-3

Impacted ampullary stone. Unusual peanut-shaped configuration *(arrow)*.

Suggested Reading

Cohen SM, Kurtz AB. Biliary sonography. *Radiol Clin North Am* 1991;29:1171.

Mirizzi Syndrome

KEY FACTS

- Extrinsic right-sided compression of the common hepatic duct resulting from inflammation associated with an impacted stone in the cystic duct or the neck of the gallbladder
- Symptoms of acute cholecystitis and jaundice
- Can result in inflammatory or mechanical obstruction of the biliary tree
- CT shows an inflammatory mass in the porta hepatis and may identify the cystic duct stone
- Preoperative radiographic diagnosis is difficult but critical, lest the surgeon inadvertently ligate the common hepatic duct (mistaking it for the cystic duct)

FIGURE 20-4

Mirizzi syndrome. Endoscopic retrograde cholangiopancreatography (ERCP) demonstrates a stone *(white arrows)* that has penetrated into the common hepatic duct, causing obstruction with stenosis. The shrunken gallbladder is opacified by a cholecysto-biliary fistula *(black arrows)*. The cystic duct was not identified at surgery. (From Becker CD, Hassler H, Terrier F. Preoperative diagnosis of the Mirizzi syndrome: limitations of sonography and computed tomography. *AJR* 1984;143:591, with permission.)

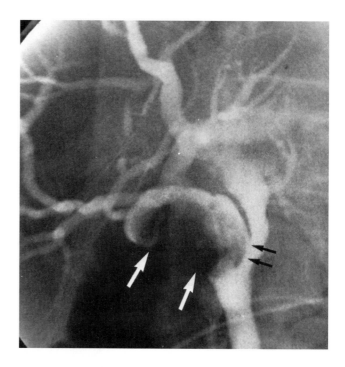

FIGURE 20-5

Mirizzi syndrome. Transhepatic cholangiogram shows a filling defect in the common hepatic duct *(arrows)* due to a large gallstone penetrating from the cystic duct. At surgery, this jaundiced patient had a fistula from the neck of the gallbladder to the common hepatic duct. (From Cruz FO, Barriga P, Tocornal J, et al. Radiology of the Mirizzi syndrome: diagnostic importance of the transhepatic cholangiogram. *Gastrointest Radiol* 1983;8:249, with permission.)

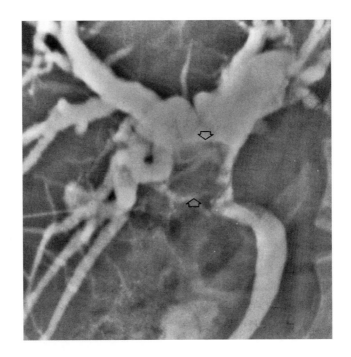

Suggested Reading

Becker CD, Hassler H, Terrier F. Preoperative diagnosis of the Mirizzi syndrome: limitations of sonography and computed tomography. *AJR* 1984;143:591.

Biliary Atresia

KEY FACTS

- Most common cause of persistent neonatal jaundice
- Probably develops postpartum as a complication of a chronic inflammatory process that causes ductal luminal obliteration
- Radionuclide scans show rapid hepatic activity, but delayed clearance from the cardiac blood pool and no visualization of bowel on delayed images taken at 24 hours (this appearance can also be seen with neonatal hepatitis or biliary tract hypoplasia)
- Portoenterostomy can result in a cure rate of 90% if the diagnostic is made before 2 months of age (before liver damage progresses to an advanced stage)
- After 3 months of age, the surgical success rate drops to <20%

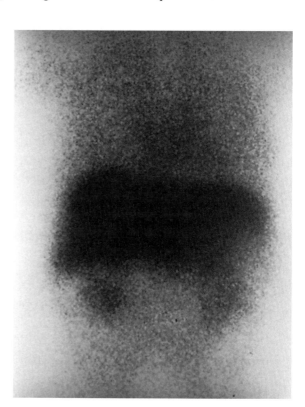

FIGURE 20-6
Biliary atresia. Sulfur-colloid scan shows uptake throughout the liver but no excretion of radionuclide into the gastrointestinal tract. The activity below the liver is in the kidneys. Some liver dysfunction and poor excretion of radionuclide are indicated by the persistent vascular activity in the heart. (From Gore RM, Levine MS, Laufer I, eds. *Textbook of gastrointestinal radiology.* Philadelphia: WB Saunders, 1994, with permission.)

Suggested Reading
Larsen CR, Scholz FJ, Wise RE. Diseases of the biliary ducts. *Semin Roentgenol* 1976;11:259.

Biliary Stricture

KEY FACTS

- Almost all benign strictures are related to previous biliary tract surgery
- Infrequently, blunt abdominal trauma causes torsion injury to the common bile duct
- Smooth, concentric narrowing of the bile duct
- Unlike malignant lesions, benign strictures usually involve long segments and have a gradual transition without complete obstruction

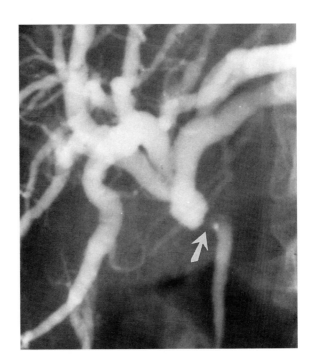

FIGURE 20-7
Biliary stricture. Narrowing of the common bile duct *(arrow)* related to previous biliary tract surgery.

Suggested Reading

Menuck L, Amberg J. The bile ducts. *Radiol Clin North Am* 1976;14:499.

Cholangitis

PRIMARY SCLEROSING CHOLANGITIS

KEY FACTS

- Rare chronic cholestatic liver disease of unknown etiology that is characterized by patchy progressive fibrosis of the biliary tree
- 70% of patients are male; 70% are under age 45 at the time of diagnosis; and 70% have ulcerative colitis
- Multiple segmental strictures involving both the intrahepatic and extrahepatic bile ducts alternating with normal or less involved duct segments produce the classic beaded appearance on cholangiography
- Diverticular outpouchings and a pruned tree appearance due to obliteration of peripheral ducts are characteristic features
- CT and ultrasound show concentric or asymmetric thickening of the walls of larger bile ducts (also gallstones, seen in 25% of cases)

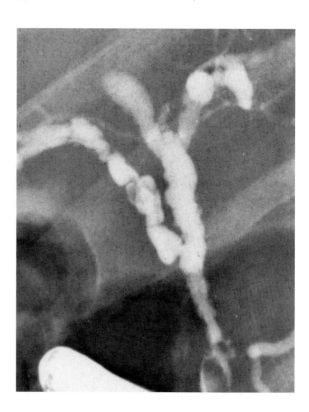

FIGURE 20-8
Primary sclerosing cholangitis. Beaded cholangiographic appearance in a patient with chronic ulcerative colitis.

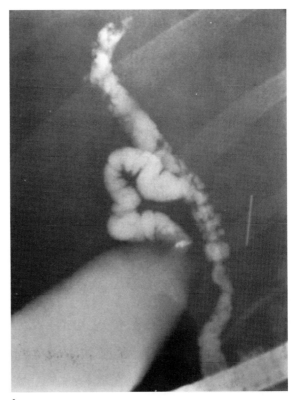

A

FIGURE 20-9
Primary sclerosing cholangitis.
A: Extensive complex band
strictures with diverticula involving
the common hepatic and bile ducts.
Note the normal valves of Heister
in the cystic duct. **B:** Confluent
strictures, several centimeters in
length, involve the intrahepatic
ducts and the common hepatic duct.
The diminished arborization of the
intrahepatic ducts results in a
classic pruned-tree appearance.
(From MacCarty RL, LaRusso NF,
Wiesner RH, et al. Primary
sclerosing cholangitis: findings on
cholangiography and
pancreatography. *Radiology*
1983;149:39, with permission.)

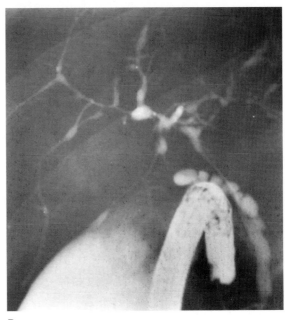

B

Suggested Reading
MacCarty RL, LaRusso NF, Wiesner RH, et al. Primary sclerosing cholangitis: findings on
cholangiography and pancreatography. *Radiology* 1983;149:39.

OBSTRUCTIVE CHOLANGITIS

KEY FACTS

- Bacterial infection related to biliary obstruction (usually benign) causing bile stasis
- Acute symptoms of right upper quadrant pain, chills, fever, and jaundice
- Purulent bile may be identified as echogenic material within involved ducts on ultrasound or as high-density intraductal material on CT
- Repeated episodes of infection may lead to duct strictures, peripheral attenuation of intrahepatic bile ducts, and biliary cirrhosis (simulates primary sclerosing cholangitis, though an obstructive cause such as stones or postoperative stricture is usually clinically or radiographically obvious)

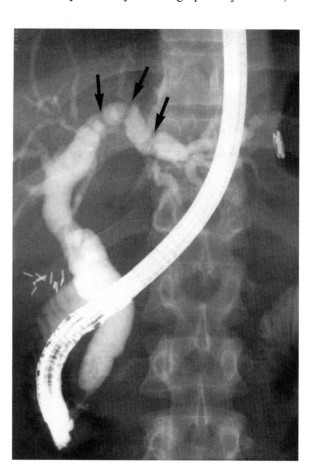

FIGURE 20-10

Cryptosporidiosis cholangitis in AIDS. Beading of the proximal left hepatic duct is caused by strictures *(arrows)*, as is narrowing and irregularity of ductal branches. The common hepatic and common bile ducts are irregular and dilated to the level of the ampulla. (From Teixidor HS, Godwin TA, Ramirez EA: Cryptosporidiosis of the biliary tract in AIDS. *Radiology* 1991;180:51, with permission.)

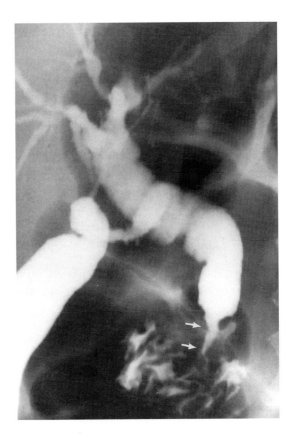

FIGURE 20-11

Cytomegalovirus cholangitis in AIDS. Fixed, irregular narrowing of the distal 2 cm of the common bile duct *(arrows)* with associated dilatation and irregularity of the more proximal portions of the biliary tree. (From Teixidor HS, Honig CL, Norsoph E, et al. Cytomegalovirus infection of the alimentary canal. Radiologic findings with pathologic correlation. *Radiology* 1987;163:317, with permission.)

Suggested Reading

Teixidor HS, godwin TA, Ramirez EA: Cryptosporidiosis of the biliary tract in AIDS. *Radiology* 1991;180:51.

RECURRENT PYOGENIC CHOLANGITIS (ORIENTAL CHOLANGIOHEPATITIS)

KEY FACTS

- Major cause of acute abdomen in Asia
- Recurrent attacks of right upper quadrant pain, fever, chills, and jaundice
- Multiple soft pigmented stones form within markedly dilated intrahepatic and extrahepatic biliary ducts (due to bile stasis and recurrent infection with gram-negative bacteria)
- CT and ultrasound demonstrate stones and sludge within dilated bile ducts (especially involving the lateral segment of the left lobe)
- Decreased arborization and abrupt tapering of intrahepatic bile ducts on cholangiography

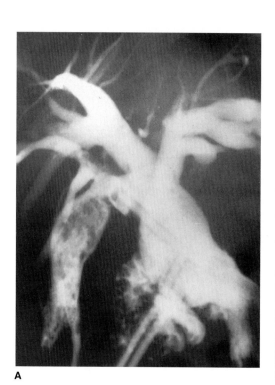

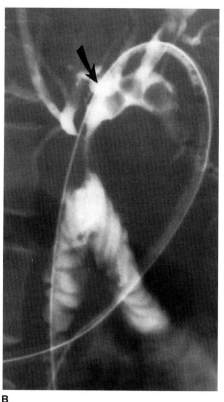

A

B

FIGURE 20-12 Recurrent pyogenic cholangitis (Oriental cholangiohepatitis). **A:** Numerous calculi within a dilated right intrahepatic duct. **B:** In a different patient with recurrent cholangitis after choledochal-jejunostomy, there are multiple calculi *(arrow)* within the left ductal system. (From Kerlan RK, Pogany AC, Goldberg HI, et al. Radiologic intervention in oriental cholangiohepatitis. *AJR* 1985;145:809, with permission.)

Suggested Reading
Kerlan RK, Pogany AC, Goldberg HI, et al. Radiologic intervention in Oriental cholangio-hepatitis. *AJR* 1985;145:809.

Clonorchiasis

KEY FACTS

- Chinese liver fluke (*Clonorchis sinensis*) that is ingested by humans who eat uncooked fish in endemic areas in Asia
- Larvae migrate up the biliary tree (especially the peripheral branches), where they burrow into the duct walls and incite an inflammatory reaction
- Combination of biliary stricture, stone formation, and conglomeration of the worms can result in obstructive jaundice
- In addition to narrowing of the bile ducts, there may be multiple crescent-shaped filling defects and communicating abscess cavities
- In endemic areas, *Ascaris lumbricoides* can cross the sphincter of Oddi from the duodenum and cause partial or complete obstruction of bile ducts, with resultant cholangitis, cholecystitis, and stone formation

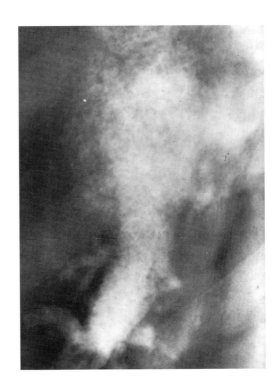

FIGURE 20-13
Clonorchiasis. Multiple filling defects in the biliary system, many of which represent coexistent calculi that are often seen in this condition.

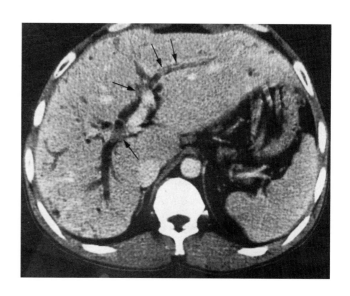

FIGURE 20-14

Clonorchiasis. Post-contrast CT scan shows high-attenuation casts *(arrows)* that presumably represent aggregates of the liver flukes within dilated intrahepatic ducts. (From Lim JH. Radiologic findings of clonorchiasis. *AJR* 1990;155:1001, with permission.)

Suggested Reading

Lim JH. Radiologic findings in clonorchiasis. *AJR* 1990;155:1001.

Choledochal Cyst

KEY FACTS

- Congenital cystic or fusiform dilatation that primarily involves the extrahepatic portions of the bile duct
- Typically associated with localized constriction of the distal common bile duct
- Classic clinical triad of upper abdominal pain, mass, and jaundice (only occurs in 30% of cases)
- Increased risk of cholangiocarcinoma
- CT and ultrasound demonstrate a fluid-filled structure beneath the porta hepatis that is separate from the gallbladder and communicates with the biliary tree
- Abrupt change of caliber where the dilated segment joins the normal duct

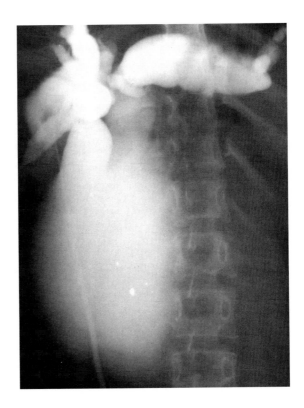

FIGURE 20-15

Choledochal cyst. The intrahepatic bile ducts are also involved in the generalized dilatation of the biliary system.

FIGURE 20-16

Choledochal cyst. Longitudinal sonogram to the right of the midline shows a large choledochal cyst *(C)* located in the region of the hilum of the liver and extending down to the area of the pancreatic head. Note the dilated proximal common hepatic duct *(arrow)* branching off from the cystic mass and dilated central intrahepatic ducts *(arrowhead)*. *K*, kidney. (From Han BK, Babcock DS, Gelfand MH. Choledochal cyst with bile duct dilatation: sonography and 99mTc IDA cholescintigraphy. *AJR* 1981;136:1075, with permission.)

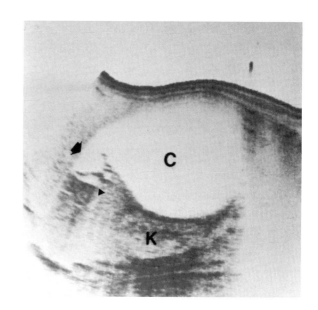

FIGURE 20-17

Choledochal cyst. CT scan shows a 15-cm choledochal cyst. (From Araki T, Itai Y, Tasaka A. Computed tomography of choledochal cyst. *AJR* 1980;135:1981, with permission.)

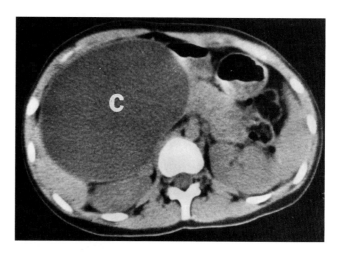

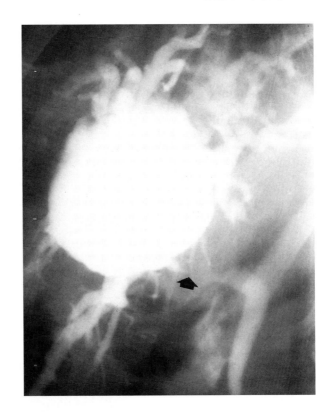

FIGURE 20-18
Choledochal cyst. Localized
constriction *(arrow)* separates
the cyst from the normal-caliber
distal duct.

Suggested Reading

Han BH, Babcock DS, Gelfand MH. Choledochal cyst with bile duct dilatation: sonography
    and 99mTc IDA cholescintigraphy. *AJR* 1981;136:1075.

Caroli's Disease

KEY FACTS

- Rare condition in which there is segmental saccular dilatation of intrahepatic bile ducts throughout the liver (cavernous ectasia of the biliary tree)

- The dilated cystic segments contain bile and communicate freely with the biliary tree and with each other

- Autosomal recessive but frequently not discovered until young adulthood

- About 80% have associated medullary sponge kidney

- No cirrhosis or portal hypertension (unlike congenital hepatic fibrosis)

- Complications include stone formation within the dilated intrahepatic ducts, recurrent cholangitis, liver abscesses, and increased risk of cholangiocarcinoma

- On ultrasound, multiple anechoic hepatic masses (superficially identical to polycystic disease, but in Caroli's disease careful scanning usually shows communication with the biliary tree)

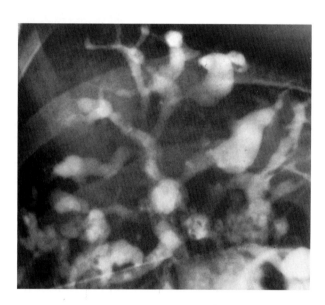

FIGURE 20-19
Caroli's disease. Segmental saccular dilatation of the intrahepatic bile ducts throughout the liver.

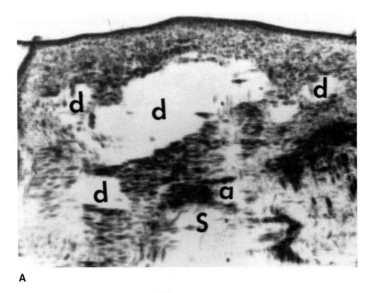

A

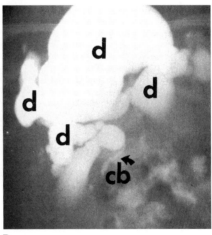

B

FIGURE 20-20

Caroli's disease. **A:** Transverse supine sonogram demonstrates the multiple dilated bile ducts *(d)* as sonolucent spaces within the liver. *s*, spine; *a*, aorta. **B:** Frontal view of a transhepatic cholangiogram in the same projection shows cystic dilatation of the distal intrahepatic ducts *(d)* with a normal-sized common bile duct *(cb)*. (From Mittelstaedt CA, Volberg FM, Fischer GJ, et al. Caroli's disease: sonographic findings. *AJR* 1980;134:585, with permission.)

Suggested Reading

Caroli J. Diseases of the intrahepatic biliary tree. *Clin Gastroenterol* 1973;2:147.

Congenital Hepatic Fibrosis

KEY FACTS

- Massive periportal fibrosis that leads to fatal liver failure and portal hypertension at an early age
- Excessive proliferation of small intrahepatic ducts that form cyst-like structures that may enlarge and simulate the cysts in Caroli's disease
- Contrast studies demonstrate a "lollipop-tree" appearance of the biliary system

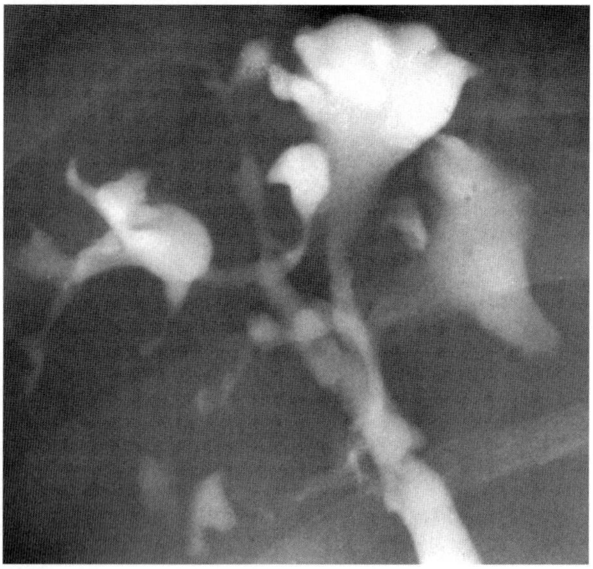

FIGURE 20-21

Congenital hepatic fibrosis. Operative cholangiogram demonstrates a lollipop-tree appearance of the biliary system. (From Unite I, Maitem A, Bagnasco SM, et al. Congenital hepatic fibrosis associated with renal tubular ectasia. *Radiology* 1973;190:565, with permission.)

Suggested Reading

Unite I, Maitem A, Bagnasco SM, et al. Congenital hepatic fibrosis associated with renal tubular ectasia. *Radiology* 1973;190:565.

Choledochocele

KEY FACTS

- Cystic dilatation of the intraduodenal portion of the common bile duct
- On upper GI series, a well-defined, smooth duodenal filling defect in the region of the papilla
- On cholangiography, the bulbous terminal portion of the common bile duct fills with contrast and projects into the duodenal lumen (separated from contrast in the duodenal lumen by a radiolucent membrane) and mimics a ureterocele

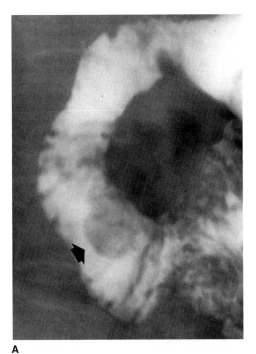 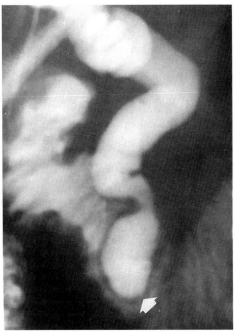

A   B

FIGURE 20-22   Choledochocele. **A:** Well-defined, smooth filling defect *(arrow)* projects into the duodenal lumen on an upper gastrointestinal series. **B:** At cholangiography, the bulbous terminal portion of the common bile duct fills with contrast and projects into the duodenal lumen *(arrow)*. It is separated from contrast in the duodenum by a radiolucent membrane.

Suggested Reading

Scholz FJ, Carrera GF, Larsen CR. The choledochocele: correlation of radiological, clinical, and pathological findings. *Radiology* 1976;118:28.

Cholangiocarcinoma

KEY FACTS

- Most commonly affects the retroduodenal or supraduodenal segments of the common bile duct
- Lesions are usually far advanced at the time of diagnosis, extending along the bile duct and spreading to regional lymph nodes
- Predisposing conditions include primary sclerosing cholangitis, choledochal cyst, congenital hepatic fibrosis, Clonorchis infection, and exposure to Thorotrast
- Klatskin tumors arising at the junction of the right and left hepatic ducts tend to grow slowly and metastasize late
- Radiographic findings include:
  a. short, well-demarcated segmental narrowing of the bile duct
  b. diffuse ductal narrowing (extensive desmoplastic response)
  c. rarely multicentric (mimicking sclerosing cholangitis)
- CT is the most sensitive modality for detecting the low-density mass, which may have a variable enhancement pattern
- Cholangiography (often requiring opacification of the ducts both from above and below) is needed to fully evaluate the extent of the tumor

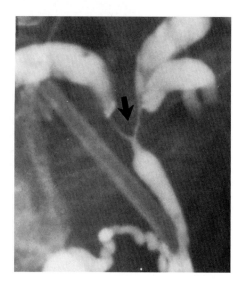

FIGURE 20-23

Cholangiocarcinoma (Klatskin tumor). Short segmental constrictions of both the right and left hepatic ducts *(arrow)*.

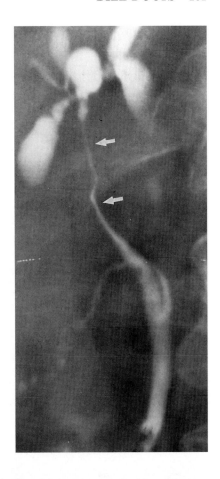

FIGURE 20-24

Cholangiocarcinoma. Severe narrowing of a long segment of the common hepatic duct *(arrows)*.

FIGURE 20-25

Cholangiocarcinoma associated with clonorchiasis. Irregular low-attenuation mass with peripheral contrast enhancement in the posterior segment of the right lobe of the liver. Note the mild diffuse dilatation of the intrahepatic bile ducts. (From Choi BI, Kim HJ, Han MC, et al. CT findings of clonorchiasis. *AJR* 1989;152:281, with permission.)

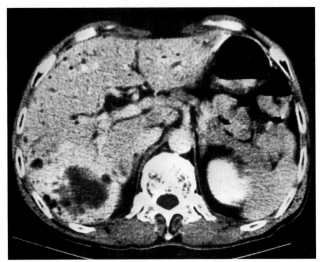

Suggested Readings

Klatskin G. Adenocarcinoma of the hepatic duct at its bifurcation within the porta hepatis: an unusual tumor with distinctive clinical and pathological features. *Am J Med* 1965;38:241.

Nichols DA, MacCarty RL, Gaffey TA. Cholangiographic evaluation of bile duct carcinoma. *AJR* 1983;141:1291.

Ampullary Carcinoma

KEY FACTS

- Small neoplasm that can appear as a polypoid mass or merely obstruct the distal end of the bile duct without a demonstrable tumor mass
- Much better prognosis than that for carcinoma of the common bile duct (5-year survival rate of 40% vs. <2%), because the localized ampullary neoplasms are more amenable to surgical resection

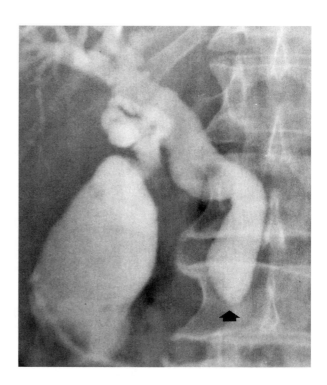

FIGURE 20-26

Ampullary carcinoma. Abrupt occlusion of the distal common bile duct *(arrow)*.

Suggested Reading

Buck JL, Elsayed AM. Ampullary tumors: radiologic-pathologic correlation. *Radiographics* 1993;13:193.

Part G
LIVER

21 Cystic Disease

Simple Cysts

KEY FACTS

- Usually of congenital, developmental origin (though some may develop after an episode of trauma or secondary to a localized inflammatory process)
- Most are asymptomatic and discovered incidentally in adulthood
- Hepatic cysts may become infected, bleed, or grow so large that they cause obstructive jaundice
- On ultrasound, a focal round or oval anechoic mass with smooth borders, thin or nondetectable walls, no septations or mural calcification, and posterior acoustic enhancement
- On CT, a sharply delineated, near-water-attenuation lesion with an imperceptible or thin smooth wall, no septations or internal structures, and no contrast enhancement
- Cysts complicated by infection or hemorrhage may have septations or internal debris (mimicking a cystic tumor)

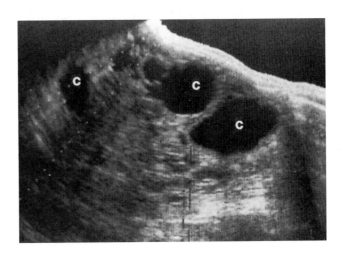

FIGURE 21-1
Simple cysts. Sagittal sonogram shows multiple anechoic masses *(c)* in the liver. (From Krebs CA, Giyanani VL, Eisenberg RL. *Ultrasound atlas of disease processes.* Norwalk, CT: Appleton & Lange, 1993, with permission.)

FIGURE 21-2
Simple cyst. A 20-cm fluid-filled mass in the right lobe of the liver displaces the abdominal contents and compresses the inferior vena cava. After aspiration and the instillation of alcohol, the cyst was virtually ablated. (From Bean WJ, Rodan BA. Hepatic cysts: treatment with alcohol. *AJR* 1985;144:237, with permission.)

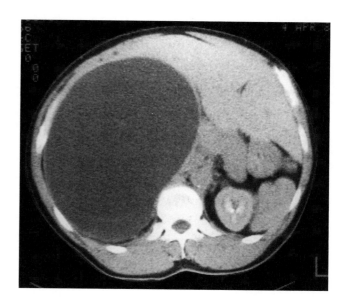

Suggested Reading

Gaines PA, Sampson M A. The prevalence and characterization of simple hepatic cysts by ultrasound examination. *Br J Radiol* 1989;62:335.

Polycystic Liver Disease

KEY FACTS

- Minimal to virtually complete replacement of the hepatic parenchyma by cystic lesions
- Occurs in about one-third of patients with adult-type polycystic kidney disease

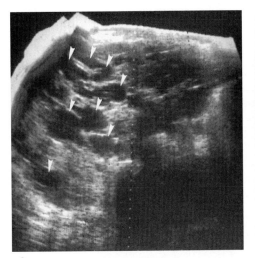

A

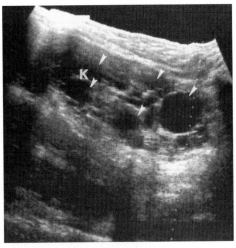

B

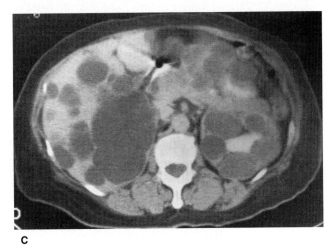

C

FIGURE 21-3   Polycystic liver disease. **A:** Transverse sonogram demonstrates multiple small anechoic masses *(arrowheads)* in the liver. **B:** Sagittal scan in the same patient shows multiple anechoic masses *(arrowheads)* in the kidney *(K)*. **C:** CT scan confirms the multiple cystic masses in the liver and kidneys. (A,B: From Krebs CA, Giyanani VL, Eisenberg RL. *Ultrasound atlas of disease processes.* Norwalk, CT: Appleton & Lange, 1993.)

Suggested Reading
Krebs CA, Giyanani VL, Eisenberg RL. *Ultrasound atlas of disease processes.* Norwalk, CT: Appleton & Lange, 1993.

22 Infectious Processes

Pyogenic Abscess

KEY FACTS

- Results from such diverse causes as:
  a. ascending biliary tract infection (especially secondary to calculi or carcinoma in the extrahepatic biliary ductal system)
  b. hematogenous spread via the portal venous system
  c. generalized septicemia (involvement of the liver via the hepatic artery circulation)
  d. direct extension from an intraperitoneal infection
  e. hepatic trauma
- On ultrasound:
  a. initially, echogenic and poorly demarcated
  b. later, variable internal echogenicity (generally less echoic) with a thickened, irregular wall
- On CT, sharply defined homogeneous mass with attenuation usually greater than a benign cyst (but lower than a solid neoplasm)
- Most have a peripheral rim or capsule of contrast enhancement (as with a necrotic neoplasm)
- Solitary abscess are usually located in the right lobe
- Gas within a low-density hepatic mass is highly suggestive of abscess

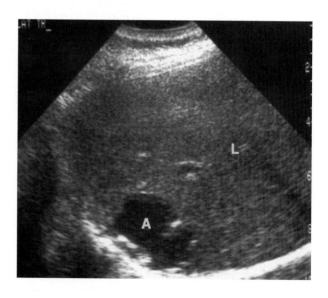

FIGURE 22-1
Pyogenic abscess. Sagittal scan shows a cystic mass *(A)* in the liver *(L)*. The mass has irregular margins and poorly defined walls and contains a mixture of low-level and high-level echoes. (From Krebs CA, Giyanani VL, Eisenberg RL. *Ultrasound atlas of disease processes.* Norwalk, CT: Appleton & Lange, 1993, with permission.)

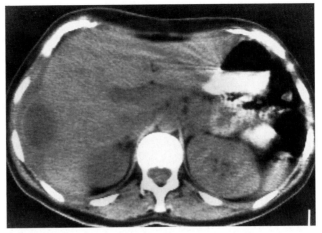

A

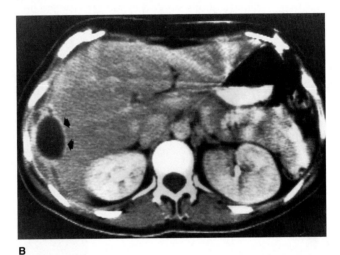

B

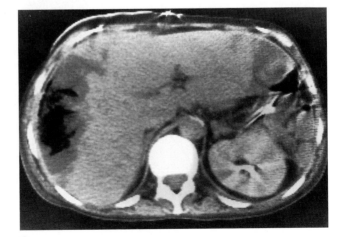

C

FIGURE 22-2
Pyogenic abscess.
A: Nonenhanced CT scan
shows a single low-
attenuation lesion with
poorly defined margins at
the periphery of the liver.
B: After contrast infusion,
there is rim enhancement
with the margins of the
abscess seen as a white line
(arrows) of higher density
than the surrounding normal
liver. **C:** In another patient,
there is a large collection of
gas in a pyogenic abscess in
the lateral aspect of the right
lobe of the liver. (From
Halvorsen RA, Korobkin M,
Foster WL, et al. The variable
appearance of hepatic
abscesses. *AJR*
1984;141:941, with
permission.)

Suggested Reading
Halvorsen RA, Korobkin M, Foster WL, et al. The variable appearance of hepatic abscesses.
AJR 1984;141:941.

Echinococcal (Hydatid) Cyst

KEY FACTS

- Tissue infection of humans caused by the larval tapeworm (dogs, sheep, cattle, and camels are the major intermediate hosts)
- On ultrasound, multiseptate complex lesion that may contain a fluid collection with a split wall or "floating membrane"
- On CT, sharply defined, near-water attenuation mass with a thin wall
- May appear multilocular with internal septations representing the walls of daughter cysts
- Complete oval or circular calcification at the periphery of a mother cyst; arc-like calcifications around daughter cysts
- Extensive dense calcifications suggest an inactive cyst, while segmental calcifications suggest cystic activity and are often considered an indication for surgery

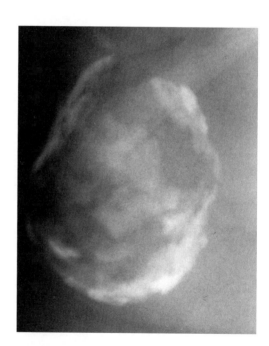

FIGURE 22-3

Calcified echinococcal cyst. Complete oval calcification is seen at the periphery of the mother cyst. Within the mother cyst are several smaller arc-like calcifications representing daughter cysts.

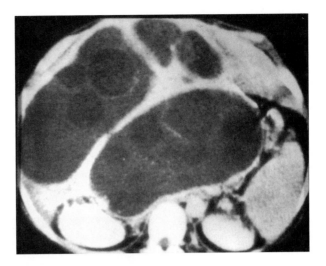

FIGURE 22-4
Echinococcal cyst. Multiple
large cysts fill a massively
enlarged liver.

Suggested Reading
Esfahani F, Rooholamini SA, Vessal K. Ultrasonography of hepatic hydatid cysts: new diagnostic signs. *J Ultrasound Med* 1988;7:443.

Amebic Abscess

KEY FACTS

- Most frequent extracolonic complication of amebiasis (occurs in about one-third of patients with amebic dysentery)
- About two-thirds are solitary
- Most often located in the posterior portion of the right lobe
- Imaging appearance similar to that of pyogenic abscess (though the patient usually is not septic and has a history of travel to an endemic area)

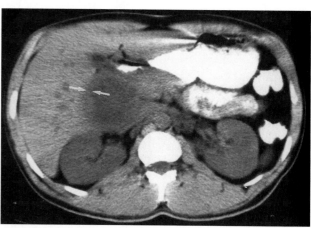

A

FIGURE 22-5

Amebic abscess.
A: Nonenhanced CT scan shows that the wall *(arrows)* has an attenuation intermediate between the center of the caudate lobe abscess and the normal hepatic parenchyma. **B:** On the enhanced scan, the wall is slightly hyperdense compared with the hepatic parenchyma. A septation *(arrowhead)* is seen medially. (From Radin DR, Ralls PW, Colletti PM, et al. CT of amebic liver abscess. *AJR* 1988;150:1297, with permission.)

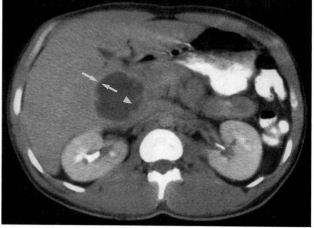

B

Suggested Reading

Radin DR, Ralls PW, Colletti PM, et al. CT of amebic liver abscess. *AJR* 1988;150:1297.

Fungal Abscess

KEY FACTS

- Uncommon condition that usually occurs in patients with compromised immune systems (leukemia, AIDS, chemotherapy, transplantation)
- Multiple small, rounded low-attenuation lesions scattered rather uniformly throughout the liver
- Central high density focus may produce a target appearance

FIGURE 22-6

Fungal abscesses. Numerous low-attenuation lesions in a massively enlarged liver, representing multiple candidal abscesses in a patient with AIDS. (From Callen PW, Filly RA, Marcus FS: Ultrasonography and computed tomography in the evaluation of hepatic microabscesses in the immunocompromised patient. *Radiology* 1980;136:433, with permission.)

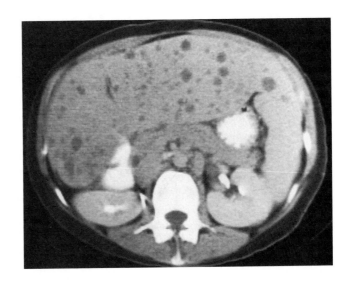

Suggested Reading

Callen PW, Filly RA, Marcus FS. Ultrasonography and computed tomography in the evaluation of hepatic microabscesses in the immunocompromised patient. *Radiology* 1980; 136:433.

23   Neoplasms

Hemangioma of the Liver

KEY FACTS

- Most common benign tumor of the liver (1% to 10% incidence)
- Usually single, small, and asymptomatic (found incidentally at surgery or autopsy or during an unrelated imaging procedure)
- On ultrasound, virtually pathognomonic appearance of a highly echogenic focus superimposed on a background of normal liver parenchyma
- On precontrast CT, a well-circumscribed low-attenuation mass
- After bolus contrast injection, the classic pattern is peripheral enhancement that advances centripetally so that the central area of low density becomes progressively smaller and the lesion eventually becomes isodense (or even hyperdense) to the liver parenchyma
- Large tumors with central areas of necrosis, fibrosis, or scar may not completely "fill in" with contrast material
- On MRI, marked hyperintensity on T2-weighted images (on T1-weighted images, contrast enhancement pattern is similar to that on CT)
- Tagged blood pool radionuclide scans demonstrate a defect in early images that shows prolonged and persistent "filling in" on delayed scans

FIGURE 23-1
Hemangioma. Transverse sonogram shows a characteristic hyperechoic mass containing homogeneous echoes *(arrows). L,* liver. (From Krebs CA, Giyanani VL, Eisenberg RL. *Ultrasound atlas of disease processes.* Norwalk, CT: Appleton & Lange, 1993, with permission.)

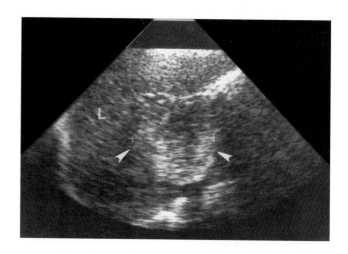

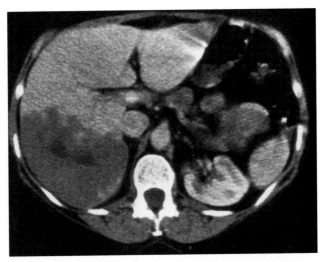

A

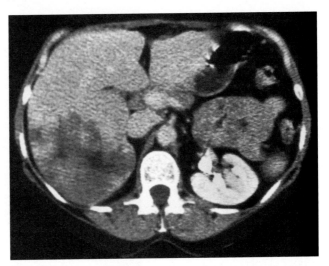

B

FIGURE 23-2
Hemangioma. **A:** Initial scan after a bolus of contrast material demonstrates a large low-attenuation lesion in the posterior segment of the right lobe. **B,C:** Delayed scans show progressive enhancement of the lesion until it becomes nearly isodense with the normal hepatic parenchyma.

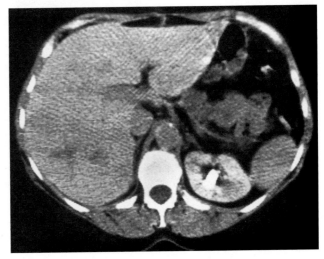

C

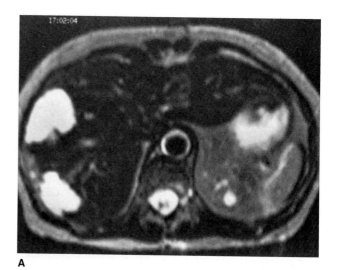

A

B

C

FIGURE 23-3

Hemangioma. **A:** The lesions are markedly hyperintense on this T2-weighted scan. **B:** Immediately after contrast administration, there is peripheral enhancement similar to that seen on CT. **C:** Ten minutes later, the lesions have completely filled in. The upper pole *(arrow)* of the left kidney contains a small cyst that is not enhanced, though it was markedly hyperintense on the T2-weighted image **(A)**. (From Gore RM, Levine, MS, Laufer I, eds. *Handbook of gastrointestinal radiology.* Philadelphia: WB Saunders, 1994, with permission.)

Suggested Reading

Freeny PC, Marks WM. Hepatic hemangioma: dynamic bolus CT. *AJR* 1986;147:711.

Hepatocellular Adenoma

KEY FACTS

- Rare benign tumor that occurs almost exclusively in young women with long-term oral contraceptive use

- Generally a solitary mass that is composed entirely of hepatocytes without Kupffer's cells

- Spontaneous hemorrhage, sometimes of life-threatening proportions, is relatively common

- On ultrasound, a large, well-defined solid mass that may contain lucent areas due to necrosis or hemorrhage

- On CT, a low-attenuation or almost isodense mass with variable degree of enhancement (spontaneous acute hemorrhage produces a central focus of increased attenuation)

FIGURE 23-4

Hepatocellular adenoma. Transverse sonogram shows a well-defined, solid echogenic mass *(M)* with a hypoechoic halo *(arrow)*. L, liver. (From Krebs CA, Giyanani VL, Eisenberg RL. *Ultrasound atlas of disease processes.* Norwalk, CT: Appleton & Lange, 1993, with permission.)

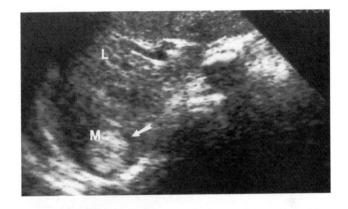

FIGURE 23-5

Hepatocellular adenoma. Large low-attenuation mass within the liver. Note the area of higher attenuation *(arrows)*, which represented a blood clot, along the posterior aspect of the lesion.

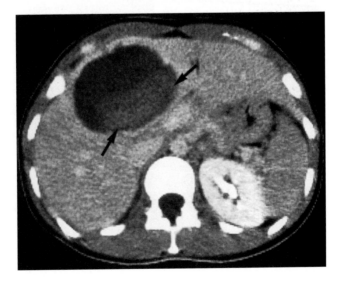

Suggested Reading
Mathieu D, Bruneton JN, Drouilard J, et al. Hepatic adenomas and focal nodular hyperplasia. Dynamic CT study. *Radiology* 1986;160:53.

Focal Nodular Hyperplasia

KEY FACTS

- Benign tumor-like condition characterized by a central stellate fibrous scar with peripheral radiating septa that divide the mass into lobules
- More common in women (85%) but not associated with oral contraceptive use (unlike hepatocellular adenoma)
- Typically occurs in a subcapsular location (infrequently deep in the hepatic parenchyma)
- On ultrasound, a well-demarcated solid mass of variable echogenicity (80% solitary)
- On CT, nonspecific low-attenuation mass that often demonstrates substantial enhancement
- Large central scar may appear on CT as a relatively low-density stellate area within a generally enhancing mass (also may be seen in some hepatic adenomas or hepatocellular carcinomas)
- On MRI, homogeneous isointense lesion with a central scar that appears hypointense on T1-weighted images and hyperintense on T2-weighted scans (in hepatocellular carcinoma, the scar has low signal intensity on T2)
- Unlike hepatocellular adenoma and other liver tumors, focal nodular hyperplasia contains technetium-avid Kupffer's cells and thus appears normal on a radionuclide liver scan
- Hot spots in the lesion (increased number of Kupffer's cells seen in 10% of cases) may be a specific feature

FIGURE 23-6
Focal nodular hyperplasia. The hyperechoic mass (between the *cursor marks*) has a central scar *(arrows)* and was found in an otherwise normal liver. The middle hepatic vein *(V)* is displaced. (From Marn CS, Bree RL, Silver TM. Ultrasonography of the liver: technique and focal and diffuse disease. *Radiol Clin North Am* 1991;29:1151, with permission.)

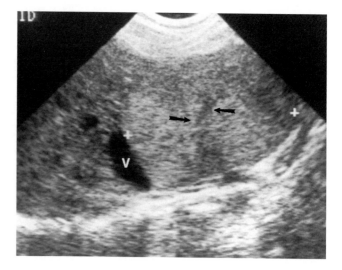

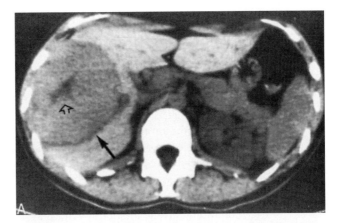

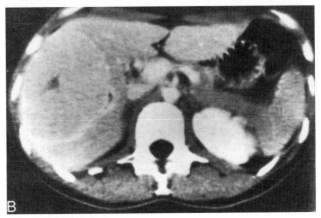

FIGURE 23-7

Focal nodular hyperplasia.
A: Noncontrast scan shows a low-attenuation lesion *(solid arrow)* with a single central spiculated area of further hypodensity *(open arrow).*
B: After bolus contrast injection, the lesion becomes slightly hyperdense compared with the normal liver. (From Gore RM, Levine MS, Laufer I, ed. *Textbook of gastrointestinal radiology.* Philadelphia: WB Saunders, 1994, with permission.)

Suggested Reading

Welch TJ, Sheedy PF, Johnson CM, et al. Radiographic characteristics of benign liver tumors: focal nodular hyperplasia and hepatic adenoma. *Radiographics* 1985;5:673

Hepatocellular Carcinoma (Hepatoma)

KEY FACTS

- In the United States, generally occurs after age 70 in patients with underlying diffuse hepatocellular disease (especially alcoholic or postnecrotic cirrhosis; hemochromatosis)

- Extremely common in Africa and Asia, where the tumor is far more aggressive, is often associated with parasitic infestation, and may account for up to one-third of all malignancies

- Unlike metastases, hepatomas:
  a. tend to be solitary or produce a small number of lesions
  b. commonly invade the portal venous system

- On ultrasound, small tumors (<3 cm) often appear hypoechoic and are associated with posterior acoustic enhancement, whereas large tumors (>3 cm) may be hyperechoic or have a mosaic or mixed pattern

- On CT, a large hypodense mass with central areas of lower attenuation (corresponding to frequent tumor necrosis)

- On contrast scans, the tumor appears hyperdense in nonnecrotic areas and there is intense rim enhancement of any surrounding capsule

- Detection of hepatocellular carcinoma on a background of cirrhosis and regenerating nodules may pose a diagnostic challenge, but an elevated level of serum alpha-fetoprotein (seen in 90%) is highly suggestive

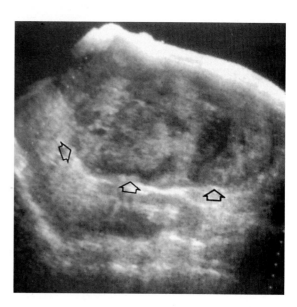

FIGURE 23-8

Hepatocellular carcinoma. Complex mass *(arrows)* with a large echogenic component.

FIGURE 23-9
Hepatocellular carcinoma. Huge low-attenuation liver mass with an irregular central necrotic area. There is minimal dilatation of the intrahepatic ducts in this patient with clonorchiasis. (From Choi BI, Kim HJ, Han MC, et al. CT findings of clonorchiasis. *AJR* 1989;152:281, with permission.)

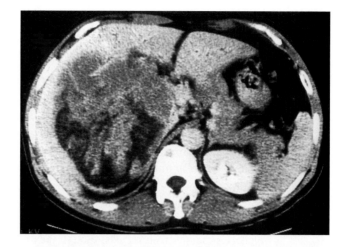

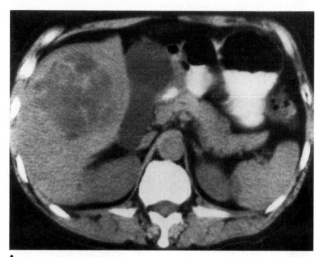

A

FIGURE 23-10
Hepatocellular carcinoma. Precontrast **(A)** and postcontrast **(B)** scans show nonuniform pattern of enhancement. (From Teefey SA, Stephens DH, James EM, et al. Computed tomography and ultrasonography of hepatoma. *Clin Radiol* 1986;37:339, with permission.)

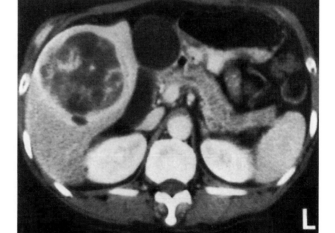

B

Suggested Reading
Teefey SA, Stephens DH, James EM, et al. Computed tomography and ultrasonography of hepatoma. *Clin Radiol* 1986;37:339.

Metastases to the Liver

KEY FACTS

- By far the most common malignant tumor involving the hepatic parenchyma
- Most common primary lesions are (in descending order) carcinomas of the colon, stomach, pancreas, breast, and lung
- Amorphous punctate deposits of calcification within the lesions suggest metastases from mucin-producing carcinomas of the gastrointestinal tract
- Variable pattern on ultrasound (no correlation between the histology of the metastasis and its sonographic appearance)
- Cystic metastases (sarcoma, melanoma, ovarian and colon carcinoma) may closely simulate benign cysts, though they often have somewhat shaggy and irregular walls
- On CT, single or more commonly multiple low-attenuation masses adjacent to normally enhancing hepatic parenchyma
- Rarely an attenuation value higher than that of liver parenchyma (diffuse calcification, recent hemorrhage, or fatty infiltration of surrounding hepatic tissue)

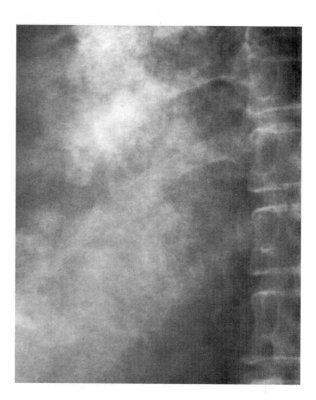

FIGURE 23-11

Metastases to the liver. Diffuse, finely granular pattern of calcification secondary to metastatic colloid carcinoma of the colon.

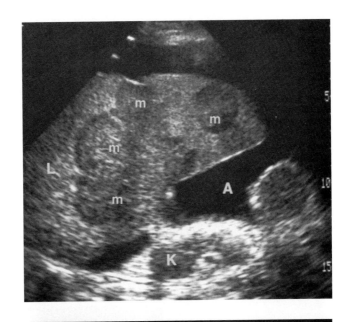

FIGURE 23-12

Metastases to the liver. Sagittal sonogram demonstrates multiple hypoechoic masses *(m)* in the liver *(L)*. Note the prominent ascitic fluid *(A)*. *K*, kidney. (From Krebs CA, Giyanani VL, Eisenberg RL. *Ultrasound atlas of disease processes.* Norwalk, CT: Appleton & Lange, 1993, with permission.)

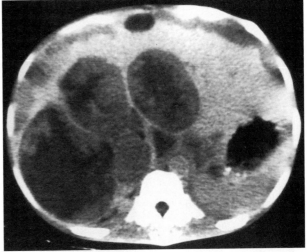

FIGURE 23-13

Metastases. CT scan shows several large low-attenuation masses that fill much of the liver. Although these lesions simulate benign cysts, their walls are somewhat shaggy and irregular.

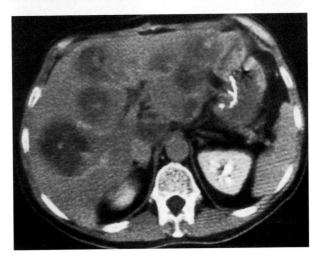

FIGURE 23-14

Multiple low-attenuation masses containing high-density centers representing calcification.

Suggested Reading

Krebs CA, Giyanani VL, Eisenberg RL. *Ultrasound atlas of disease processes.* Norwalk, CT: Appleton & Lange, 1993.

Biliary Cystadenoma/Cystadenocarcinoma

KEY FACTS

- Generally considered forms of the same disease, with cystadenocarcinoma being overtly malignant while cystadenoma merely has malignant potential
- On ultrasound, a large multicystic septated mass
- The presence of mural nodules and irregular thickening of the wall suggests malignancy
- On CT, these large, predominantly cystic tumors appear as low-attenuation lesions that are multilocular and contain numerous septations
- Neither CT nor ultrasound can reliably differentiate between these benign and malignant tumors

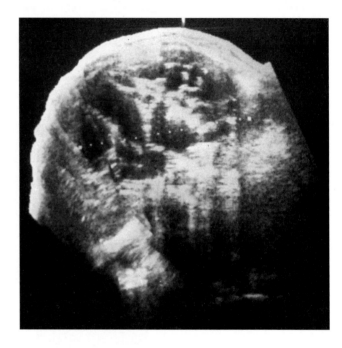

FIGURE 23-15
Biliary cystadenoma. Multiloculated liver mass. Note that the internal septa show nodular thickening and papillary excrescences. (From Choi BI, Lim JH, Han MC, et al. Biliary cystadenoma and cystadenocarcinoma: CT and sonographic findings. *Radiology* 1989;171:57, with permission.)

FIGURE 23-16
Biliary cystadenoma.
Nonenhanced scan shows a
well-defined, ovoid, low-
attenuation mass with
multiple internal septations.
Multiple calcifications
(arrows) are seen along the
wall and internal septa.
(From Choi BI, Lim JH, Han
MC, et al. Biliary
cystadenoma and
cystadenocarcinoma: CT and
sonographic findings.
Radiology 1989;171:57, with
permission.)

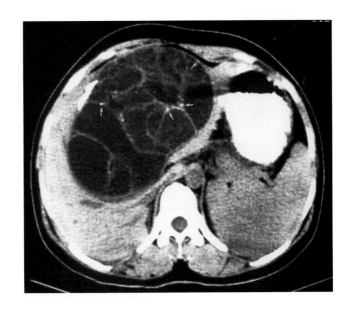

Suggested Reading

Choi BI, Lim JH, Han MC, et al. Biliary cystadenoma and cystadenocarcinoma: CT and sonographic findings. *Radiology* 1989;171:57.

Lymphoma of the Liver

KEY FACTS

- Second most common extranodal site of Hodgkin's disease
- On ultrasound, single or multiple hypoechoic masses, often with indistinct margins (may mimic the appearance of a diffuse infectious process such as candidiasis)
- CT findings include:
    a. heterogeneous liver parenchyma with ill-defined regions of decreased contrast enhancement
    b. single or multiple focal low-attenuation masses (similar to metastatic disease)
    c. diffuse lymphomatous infiltration generally is isodense and indistinguishable from normal liver (no alteration of hepatic architecture)

FIGURE 23-17

Lymphoma. This patient had rapid development of multiple focal, hypoechoic lesions. None were present in the spleen. Biopsy with cultures did not definitely determine whether this appearance reflected candidiasis or lymphoma, but the clinical course was consistent with lymphomatous involvement of the liver. (From Marn CS, Bree RL, Silver TM. Ultrasonography of the liver: technique and focal and diffuse disease. *Radiol Clin North Am* 1991;29:1151, with permission.)

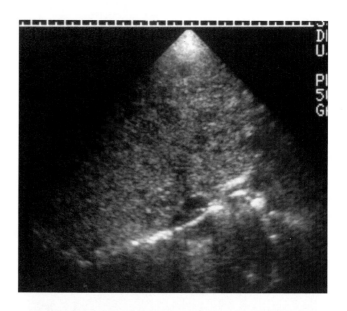

FIGURE 23-18

Lymphoma. Multiple nodules are scattered throughout the liver. (From Fishman EK, Kuhlman JE, Jones RJ. CT of lymphoma: spectrum of disease. *Radiographics* 1991;11:647, with permission.)

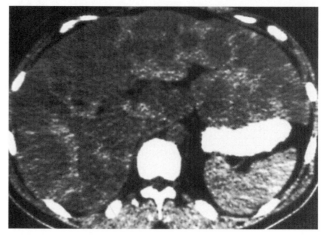

Suggested Reading

Fishman EK, Kuhlman JE, Jones RJ. CT of lymphoma: spectrum of disease. Radiographics 1991;11:647.

Hepatoblastoma

KEY FACTS

- Most common primary malignant liver neoplasm in childhood
- Usually develops within the first 3 years of life and is very aggressive (often metastasizing to lung at the time of diagnosis)
- On ultrasound, a hyperechoic mass that may show acoustic shadowing secondary to intratumoral calcification
- Hypoechoic or cystic areas within the tumor may reflect areas of hemorrhage or necrosis
- Intense neovascularity of the tumor is associated with high Doppler frequency shifts
- On CT, a low-attenuation mass with variable contrast enhancement

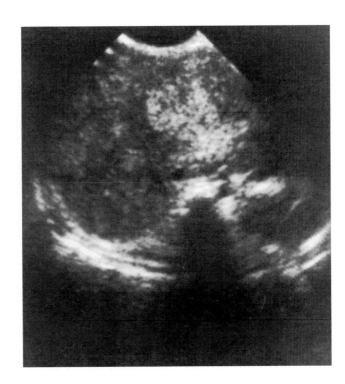

FIGURE 23-19
Hepatoblastoma. Transverse sonogram shows the echogenic mass. (From Gedgaudas-McClees RK, ed. *Handbook of gastrointestinal imaging.* New York: Churchill Livingstone, 1987, with permission.)

Suggested Reading

Dachman AH, Parker RL, Ros PR, et al. Hepatoblastoma: a radiologic-pathologic correlation in 50 cases. *Radiology* 1987;164:15.

Hemangioendothelioma

KEY FACTS

- Most common hepatic lesion producing symptoms during infancy (vast majority of these tumors present before 6 months of age)
- Generally benign (rare reports of distant metastases)
- Extensive arteriovenous shunting within the lesion may lead to high-output congestive heart failure
- On ultrasound, a complex mass containing large anechoic sinusoids and associated with prominent draining veins (reflecting the hypervascular nature of the lesion)
- On CT, a well-demarcated mass of decreased attenuation that shows early peripheral enhancement and may become completely isodense on delayed scans

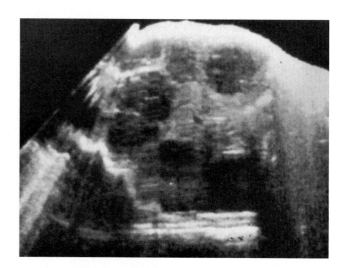

FIGURE 23-20
Hemangioendothelioma. Sagittal sonogram shows multiple discrete, hypoechoic solid masses. (From Dachman AH, Lichtenstein JE, Friedman AC, et al. Infantile hemangioendothelioma of the liver: a radiological-pathologic-clinical correlation. *AJR* 1983;140:1091, with permission.)

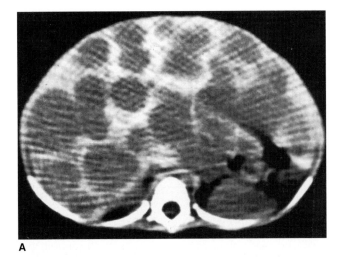

A

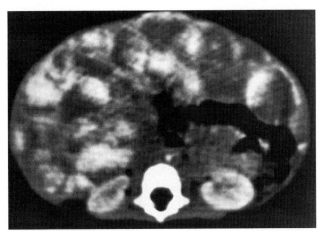

B

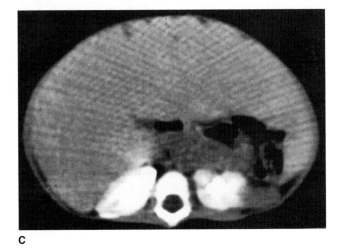

C

FIGURE 23-21

Hemangioendothelioma.
A: On the noncontrast scan, multiple rounded hypodense masses are seen throughout the liver. **B:** Immediately after contrast administration, extensive patchy enhancement is visible.
C: Delayed postcontrast scan shows that all the tumors have become isodense with the surrounding liver. (From Lucaya J, Enique G, Amat L, et al. Computed tomography of infantile hepatic hemangioendothelioma. *AJR* 1985;144:821, with permission.)

Suggested Reading

Dachman AH, Lichtenstein JE, Friedman AC, et al. Infantile hemangioendothelioma of the liver. *AJR* 1983;140:1091.

24 Other Disorders

Budd-Chiari Syndrome

- Obstruction of hepatic venous outflow at the level of the intrahepatic venules, the hepatic veins, or the suprahepatic segment of the inferior vena cava
- Rare condition that is associated with hypercoagulability states, oral contraceptives, pregnancy, invasive tumors, and congenital webs
- On CT, enlarged liver with diffusely decreased attenuation (presumably due to congestion of the hepatic parenchyma)
- "Flip-flop" pattern of contrast enhancement (also seen with congestive heart failure and constrictive pericarditis, in which there is also marked dilation of the inferior vena cava and hepatic veins due to backward transmission of elevated central pressure)

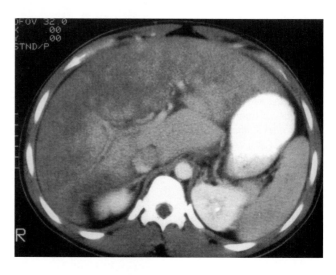

FIGURE 24-1   Budd-Chiari syndrome. Contrast scan of a woman with a coagulation disorder and hepatic vein thrombosis shows the characteristic mosaic pattern of peripheral low attenuation in both the right and left hepatic lobes. The liver is enlarged with relatively marked hypertrophy of the caudate lobe, which has a uniform attenuation. (From Foley WD, Jochem RJ. Computed tomography: focal and diffuse liver disease. *Radiol Clin North Am* 1991;29:1213, with permission.)

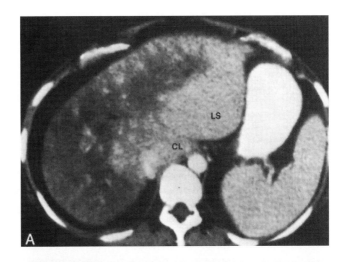

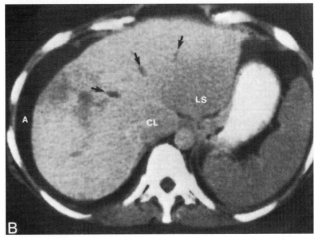

FIGURE 24-2

Budd-Chiari syndrome. Classic flip-flop pattern of hepatic contrast enhancement. **A:** Initially, the normally enhancing central part of the liver [including the caudate lobe *(CL)* and part of the lateral segment of the left lobe *(LS)*] appears hyperdense relative to the periphery of the liver, which enhances more slowly. **B:** Later, as the contrast material washes out centrally and accretes peripherally, the central region appears relatively hypodense. Note the thrombus in the hepatic veins *(arrows)*. *A*, ascites. (From Gore RM, Levine MS, Laufer I, eds. *Textbook of gastrointestinal radiology.* Philadelphia: WB Saunders, 1994, with permission.)

Suggested Reading

Foley WD, Jochem RJ. Computed tomography. Focal and diffuse liver disease. *Radiol Clin North Am* 1991;29:1213.

Cirrhosis

KEY FACTS

- Chronic liver disease characterized by diffuse parenchymal destruction, fibrosis, and nodular regeneration with distortion of the normal hepatic architecture

- In the United States, usually secondary to alcohol abuse

- Other causes include chronic viral hepatitis, schistosomiasis and other parasitic diseases, toxic agents (drugs, iron-overload), biliary obstruction, and a variety of vascular, nutritional, and hereditary disorders

- The liver is initially enlarged, but eventually becomes shrunken with a nodular surface

- Hypertrophy of the caudate lobe and shrinkage of the right lobe (caudate to right lobe ratio > 0.65 on transverse images)

- Extrahepatic signs include portal hypertension, splenomegaly, and ascites

- On ultrasound, generalized increase in echogenicity associated with decreased beam penetration and poor depiction of the intrahepatic vessels (due to fatty infiltration and fibrosis)

- In addition to the findings described above, CT may demonstrate fatty infiltration, regenerating nodules, increased density of mesenteric fat, prominence of the fissures and porta hepatis, and intrahepatic arterial-portal fistulas (early opacification of the portal vein)

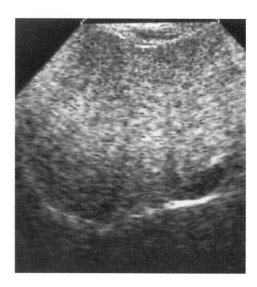

FIGURE 24-3
Cirrhosis. Diffuse increased echogenicity of the liver secondary to fibrosis.

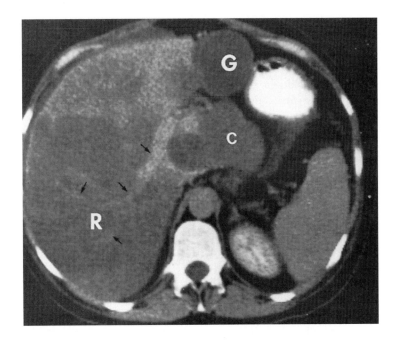

FIGURE 24-4   Cirrhosis. The right *(R)* and caudate *(c)* caudate lobes are replaced by fat to a degree that makes the density almost equal to that of the gallbladder *(G)*. The medial segment of the left hepatic lobe has a higher CT density but contains foci of low attenuation. The spleen is large and the caudate lobe is prominent. The portal vein *(arrows)* courses normally through the center of the right hepatic lobe, a sign strongly suggestive of fatty infiltration rather than tumor. (From Moss AA, Gamsu G, Genant HK, eds. *Computed tomography of the body.* Philadelphia: WB Saunders, 1992, with permission.)

Suggested Reading

Needleman L, Kurtz AB, Rifkin MD, et al. Sonography of diffuse benign liver disease: accuracy of pattern recognition and grading. *AJR* 1986;146:1011.

Fatty Infiltration

KEY FACTS

- Metabolic complication of a variety of toxic, ischemic, and infectious insults to the liver (especially alcoholic cirrhosis)
- Alcohol abuse is by far the most common cause
- Other causes include obesity, malnutrition, hyperalimentation, steroid therapy, diabetes, pancreatitis, and chemotherapy
- Fatty deposits are often transient and may completely disappear within a few weeks after withdrawal of the offending substance

DIFFUSE FORM

KEY FACTS

- On ultrasound, generally a diffuse coarse echogenicity of the liver associated with a loss of visualization of small vascular structures and poor sound penetration
- On CT, diffuse fatty infiltration causes generalized low attenuation of the liver that is much lower than that of the spleen (reversal of the normal liver-spleen density relation)
- Portal and hepatic veins commonly appear as high-attenuation structures surrounded by a background of low density caused by excessive fat (reverse of the normal pattern)

FOCAL FORM

KEY FACTS

- Discrete areas of increased echogenicity on a background of normal liver parenchyma (distinguished from metastatic disease by the lack of mass effect or displacement of portal and hepatic vein branches)
- On CT, single or multiple low-attenuation liver masses that may be difficult to differentiate from metastatic disease

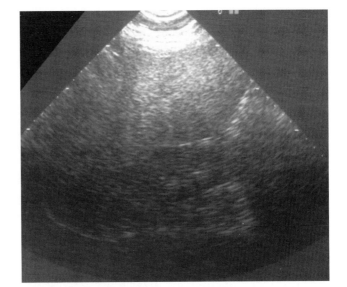

FIGURE 24-5
Fatty infiltration. Sagittal scan demonstrates a diffuse increase in echogenicity of the hepatic parenchyma with marked attenuation of the sound beam. (From Krebs CA, Giyanani VL, Eisenberg RL. *Ultrasound atlas of disease processes.* Norwalk, CT: Appleton & Lange, 1993, with permission.)

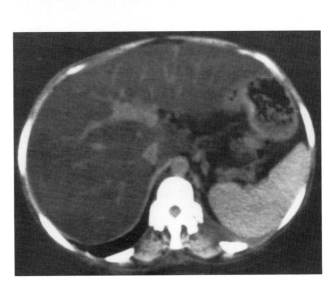

FIGURE 24-6
Fatty infiltration. In this patient with cirrhosis, the attenuation of the liver is far less than that of the spleen. The portal veins appear as high-attenuation structures surrounded by a background of low-attenuation hepatic fat.

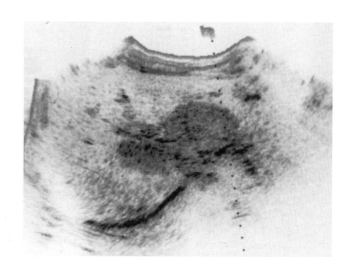

FIGURE 24-7
Focal fatty infiltration.
Longitudinal scan shows a
well-defined, densely
echogenic focus within the
liver. (From Baker MK,
Wenkler JC, Cockerill EM, et
al. Focal fatty infiltration of
the liver: diagnostic imaging.
Radiographics 1985;5:923,
with permission.)

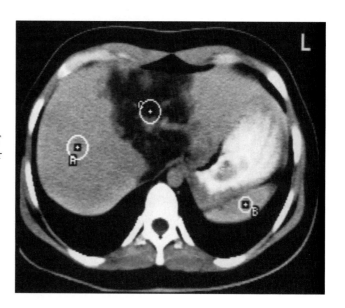

FIGURE 24-8
Focal fatty infiltration. Well-
circumscribed wedge of low
attenuation within the liver. CT
Hounsfield numbers were 4 for
the area of focal fatty
infiltration **(C)**, 80 for normal
liver **(A)**, and 83 for normal
spleen **(B)**. (From Baker MK,
Wenker JC, Cockerill EM, et
al. Focal fatty infiltration of
the liver: diagnostic imaging.
Radiographics 1985;5:923,
with permission.)

Suggested Reading

Baker MK, Wenkler JC, Cockerill EM, et al. Focal fatty infiltration of the liver: diagnostic
    imaging. *Radiographics* 1985;5:923.

Glycogen Storage Disease

KEY FACTS

- Autosomal recessive disorders of carbohydrate metabolism with various enzymatic defects
- Usually causes death in infancy, though patients may survive into adulthood with early therapy
- On CT, the excessive deposition of glycogen in the liver produces a generalized increase in hepatic attenuation
- Less commonly, the fatty infiltration that occurs in long-standing disease produces focal or diffuse low-attenuation in the liver

FIGURE 24-9

Glycogen storage disease. Diffuse increase in attenuation of the enlarged liver with prominent hepatic and portal venous structures *(arrows)*. (From Moss AA, Gamsu G, Genant HK, eds. *Computed tomography of the body.* Philadelphia: WB Saunders, 1992, with permission.)

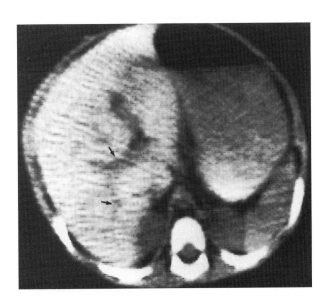

Suggested Reading

Doppman JL, Cornblath M, Dwyer AJ, et al. Computed tomography of the liver and kidneys in glycogen storage disease. *J Comput Assist Tomogr* 1982;6:67.

Hemochromatosis

KEY FACTS

- Excessive deposition of iron in body tissues with eventual fibrosis and dysfunction of the involved organs
- May be a primary inherited disorder (excessive intestinal absorption of iron) or secondary (iron medications, multiple blood transfusions, chronic hemolytic anemia)
- Substantially increased risk of hepatocellular carcinoma
- Plain radiographs show a general increase in density of the liver
- On CT, a diffuse increase in attenuation of the hepatic parenchyma, which contrasts sharply with the much lower density of the normal hepatic and portal veins
- On MRI, pronounced diffuse loss of signal intensity on T2-weighted images (most sensitive modality)

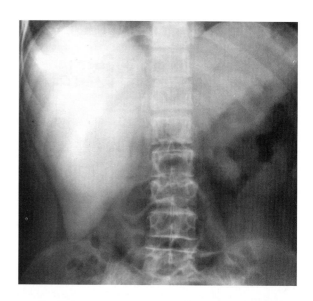

FIGURE 24-10

Hemochromatosis. Abdominal radiograph demonstrates a very dense liver shadow in the right upper quadrant caused by the parenchymal deposition of iron. (From Smith WL, Quattromani F. Radiodense liver in transfusion hemochromatosis. *AJR* 1977;128:316, with permission.)

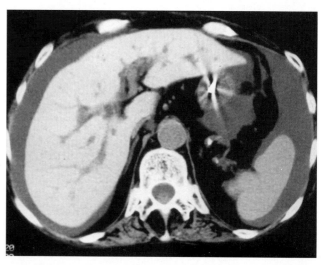

FIGURE 24-11

Hemochromatosis. Diffuse homogeneous increase in liver (and spleen) attenuation when compared with that of other soft-tissue organs. Note the hepatic and portal veins, which stand out in bold relief as low-attenuation structures against the abnormally high attenuation of the liver parenchyma. (From Foley WD, Jochem RJ. Computed tomography: focal and diffuse liver disease. *Radiol Clin North Am* 1991;29:1213, with permission.)

FIGURE 24-12

Hepatocellular carcinoma developing in hemochromatosis. The multifocal tumor *(arrows)* presents as soft-tissue-attenuation masses that appear hypodense when compared with the abnormally high attenuation of the liver parenchyma. (From Moss AA, Gamsu G, Genant HK, eds. *Computed tomography of the body.* Philadelphia: WB Saunders, 1992, with permission.)

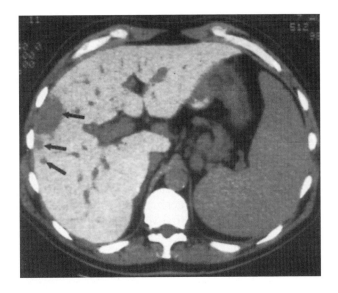

Suggested Reading

Foley WD, Jochem RJ. Computed tomography: focal and diffuse liver disease. *Radiol Clin North Am* 1991;29:1213.

Hepatitis

KEY FACTS

- Acute viral hepatitis can present a broad spectrum of clinical appearances, ranging from a mild subclinical form to fulminant liver failure
- The ultrasound appearance is frequently normal
- In *acute* hepatitis, swelling of liver cells may produce an overall decreased echogenicity of the liver associated with accentuated brightness of the portal vein walls
- In *chronic* hepatitis, the parenchymal echo pattern is coarsened because of periportal fibrosis and inflammatory cells (decreased brightness and number of portal vein radicles and an overall increase in liver echogenicity)

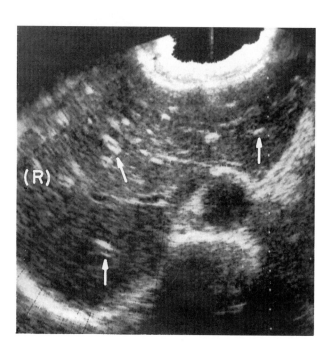

FIGURE 24-13

Acute hepatitis. Transverse scan of the right lobe of the liver shows an overall decrease in the echo pattern. Note that the portal vein radicle walls *(arrows)* are brighter than usual.

FIGURE 24-14
Chronic hepatitis.
Longitudinal scan of the right
lobe shows marked
coarsening of the liver
echoes. Note the decrease in
the brightness and number of
the portal vein radicle walls
(arrow). (From Kurtz AB,
Rubin CS, Cooper HS, et al.
Ultrasound findings in
hepatitis. *Radiology*
1980;136:717, with
permission.)

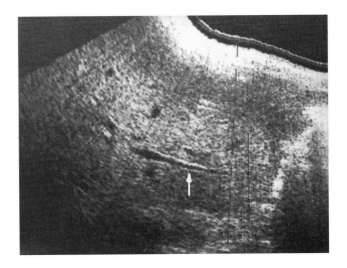

Suggested Reading

Kurtz AB, Rubin CS, Cooper HS, et al. Ultrasound findings in hepatitis. *Radiology* 1980;136:
   717.

Portal Hypertension

KEY FACTS

- Most commonly results from cirrhosis (also portal/splenic vein thrombosis, congestive heart failure, schistosomiasis)
- As portal venous pressure increases, portosystemic collaterals develop and blood is shunted away from, instead of into, the liver
- Major complications include hepatic encephalopathy and hemorrhage from varices
- Ultrasound findings include:
  a. dilatation of the portal (>13 mm), splenic (>11 mm), superior mesenteric (>12 mm), and coronary (>7 mm) veins
  b. diminished respiratory variations in the superior mesenteric and splenic veins
  c. recanalized paraumbilical veins
  d. splenomegaly
  e. collateral venous pathways (varices)
- Duplex Doppler is used to determine portal vein patency and direction of flow
- CT is superb for demonstrating the type and extent of portosystemic collaterals, which may be mistaken for lymph nodes on noncontrast scans
- In the chest, CT can distinguish varices from solid mediastinal masses

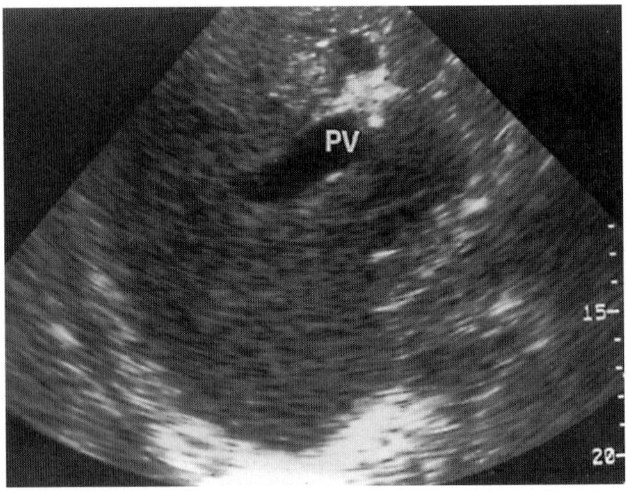

FIGURE 24-15
Portal hypertension. Sonogram shows an enlarged portal vein *(PV)* measuring >13 mm. (From Krebs CA, Giyanani VL, Eisenberg RL. *Ultrasound atlas of disease processes.* Norwalk, CT: Appleton & Lange, 1993, with permission.)

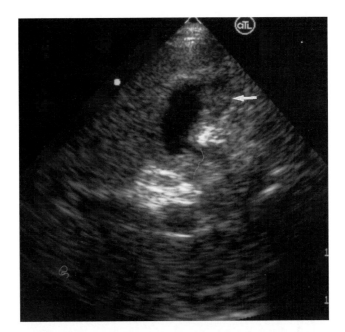

FIGURE 24-16

Portal hypertension. "Bull's-eye" ligamentum teres *(arrow)*. The central anechoic area represents the recanalized umbilical vein. (From Krebs CA, Giyanani VL, Eisenberg RL. *Ultrasound atlas of disease processes.* Norwalk, CT: Appleton & Lange, 1993, with permission.)

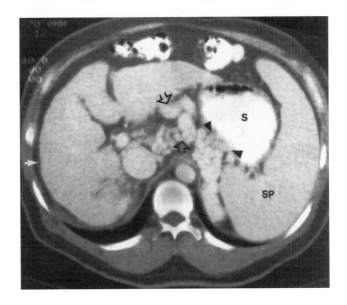

FIGURE 24-17

Portal hypertension. CT scan shows enhanced collateral veins in the gastric wall *(arrowheads)*, gastrohepatic ligament *(open arrows)*, and left retroperitoneal space. In this cirrhotic patient, note the splenomegaly and minimal ascites *(solid arrow)*. S, stomach; *SP*, spleen. (From Gore RM, Levine, MS, Laufer I, eds. *Handbook of gastrointestinal radiology.* Philadelphia: WB Saunders, 1994, with permission.)

Suggested Reading

Kane RA, Katz SG. The spectrum of sonographic findings in portal hypertension. *Radiology* 1982;142:453.

Portal Vein Thrombosis

KEY FACTS

- Most commonly the result of thrombosis secondary to preexisting portal hypertension (secondary to cirrhosis)
- Other causes include tumor invasion, intraabdominal inflammation, and trauma
- Plain radiographs may demonstrate calcification within clot or the wall of the portal vein (linear opaque density crossing the vertebral column)
- On ultrasound, echogenic material within the lumen of a dilated portal vein associated with collateral venous circulation
- On CT, low-density clot in the portal vein surrounded by peripheral enhancement

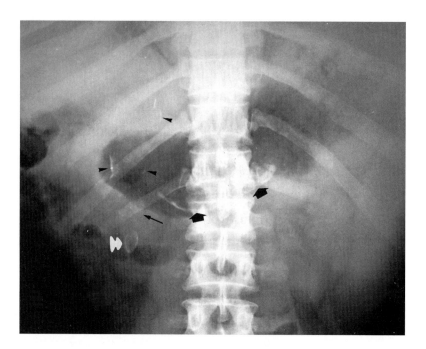

FIGURE 24-18   Portal vein thrombosis. In addition to portal vein calcification *(arrowheads)*, calcification is also seen in the walls of the splenic *(large black arrows)*, superior mesenteric *(small black arrow)* and pancreaticoduodenal veins *(white arrow)*. Note the widening of the inferior mediastinum secondary to mediastinal varices. (From Mata JH, Alegret X, Martinez A. Calcification in the portal and collateral veins wall: CT findings. *Gastrointest Radiol* 1987;12:206, with permission.)

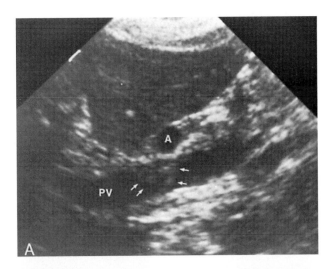

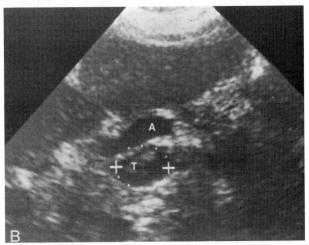

FIGURE 24-19

Portal vein thrombosis. Sagittal **(A)** and transverse **(B)** scans through the portal vein *(PV; cursors)* show the thrombus *(T)* partially occluding the lumen *(arrows)*. *A*, hepatic artery. (From Gore RM, Levine, MS, Laufer I, eds. *Handbook of gastrointestinal radiology.* Philadelphia: WB Saunders, 1994, with permission.)

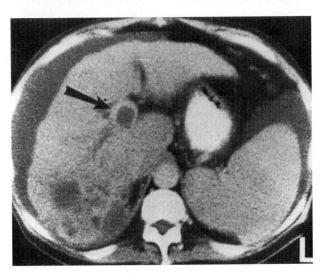

FIGURE 24-20

Portal vein thrombosis *(arrow)* in multifocal hepatocellular carcinoma. (From Teefey SA, Stephens DH, James EM, et al. Computed tomography and ultrasonography of hepatoma. *Clin Radiol* 1986;37:339, with permission.)

Suggested Reading

Mata JH, Alegret X, Martinez A. Calcification in the portal vein and collateral veins wall: CT findings. *Gastrointest Radiol* 1987;12:206.

Thorotrast

KEY FACTS

- Previously used radiographic contrast agent (thorium dioxide) that is retained in reticuloendothelial cells of the liver, spleen, and lymph nodes

- Alpha-emitting radionuclide that has been associated with the development of hepatobiliary and splenic carcinoma (especially the exceedingly rare angiosarcoma), leukemia, and aplastic anemia up to 30 years after the initial injection

- Generalized (often inhomogeneous) increased density of the liver (and spleen and lymph nodes) on both plain radiographs and CT

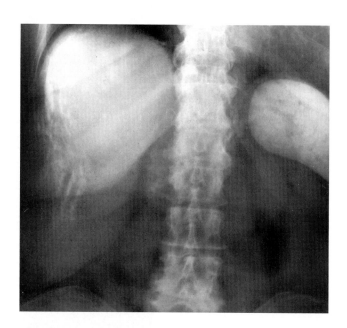

FIGURE 24-21
Thorotrast. Calcification of the liver and spleen caused by a prior injection of this radioactive contrast material.

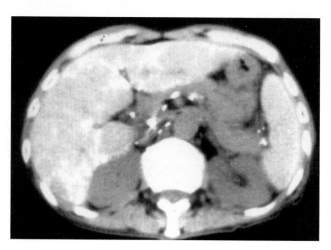

FIGURE 24-22
Thorotrast. Generalized increase in the attenuation of the liver and spleen.

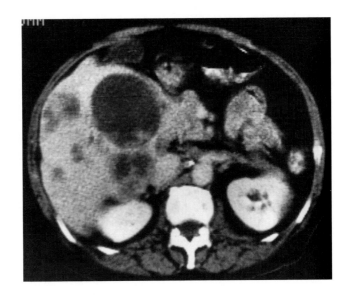

FIGURE 24-23
Angiosarcoma complicating
Thorotrast exposure.
Contrast-enhanced scan
shows multiple low-
attenuation lesions. (From
Buetow PC, Buck JL, Ros
PR, et al. Malignant vascular
tumors of the liver:
radiologic-pathologic
correlation. *Radiographics*
1994;14:153, with
permission.)

Suggested Reading

Rao BK, Brodell GK, Haaga JR. Visceral CT findings associated with Thorotrast. *J Comput Assist Tomogr* 1986:10:57.

Hepatic Trauma

KEY FACTS

- Result of blunt or penetrating abdominal trauma or a complication of surgery, percutaneous cholangiography, biopsy, portography, or biliary drainage procedures

- On CT, hematomas generally have high attenuation during the first few days, then diminish gradually over several weeks to become low-density lesions

- *Subcapsular* hematoma is a well-marginated, crescentic or lenticular collection of blood that is located at the periphery of the liver and compresses the underlying hepatic parenchyma

- *Intrahepatic* hematoma is a round or oval mass located deeper within the hepatic parenchyma

- *Parenchymal laceration* is an irregular cleft or mass of low attenuation that often extends to the periphery of the liver and may have a branching pattern superficially resembling dilated bile ducts

- *Biloma* is a low-attenuation intrahepatic or extrahepatic collection of bile due to traumatic rupture of the biliary tree

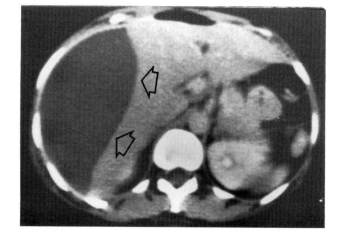

FIGURE 24-24

Subcapsular hematoma. Well-circumscribed elliptical area of low attenuation *(arrows)* in the periphery of the right lobe of the liver. The patient had sustained blunt trauma to the upper abdomen 2 weeks previously.

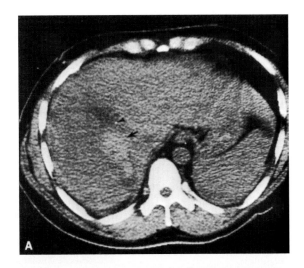

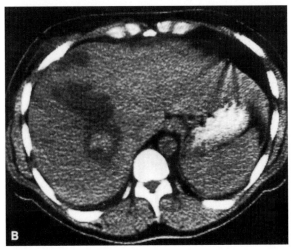

FIGURE 24-25

Intrahepatic hematoma. The patient had sustained a gunshot wound of the liver that was not appreciated at the time of laparotomy. **A:** CT scan shows the bullet fragment *(arrowhead)* in a mixed low- and high-attenuation collection. The high-attenuation area *(arrow)* represented clotted blood. **B:** One week later, the hematoma is larger and of lower attenuation. (From Margulis AR, Burhenne HJ. *Alimentary tract radiology.* St. Louis: Mosby, 1983, with permission.)

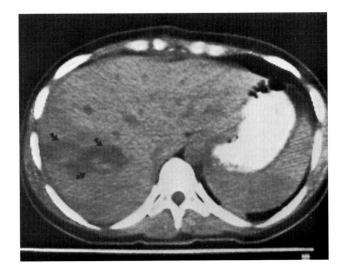

FIGURE 24-26

Hepatic laceration. CT scan after blunt trauma shows an irregular low-attenuation plane *(arrow)* passing through the right lobe of the liver. (From Margulis AR, Burhenne HJ. *Alimentary tract radiology.* St. Louis: Mosby, 1983, with permission.)

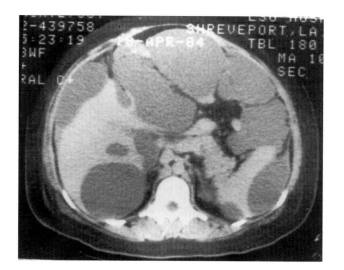

FIGURE 24-27
Biloma. Multiple intrahepatic
and extrahepatic low-
attenuation lesions after
traumatic rupture of the
biliary tree and bile
peritonitis.

Suggested Reading

Moon KL, Federle MP. Computed tomography in hepatic trauma. *AJR* 1983;141:309.

Hepatic Infarction

KEY FACTS

- Relatively uncommon because of the liver's dual blood supply (hepatic artery, portal vein) and the tolerance of hepatocytes for low levels of oxygen

- On CT, a well-circumscribed, peripheral, wedge-shaped area of low attenuation (best seen on contrast-enhanced scans)

- Similar appearance may be produced by segmental hepatic vein obstruction or by decreased portal vein flow from tumor compression or thrombus

- At times, hepatic infarcts may have a round or oval configuration and be centrally located

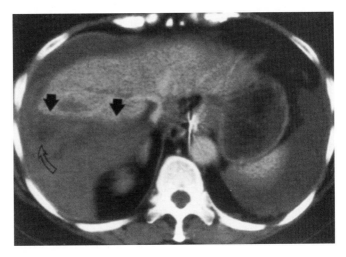

FIGURE 24-28   Infarction. Well-demarcated, wedge-shaped nonenhancing lesion in the posterior right hepatic lobe with peripheral low-attenuation components *(straight arrows)*. Peripheral low-attenuation regions *(curved arrow)* may represent focal accumulations of bile and necrotic liver. Note the presence of ascites. (From Foley WD, Jochem RJ. Computed tomography: focal and diffuse liver disease. *Radiol Clin North Am* 1991;29:1213, with permission.)

Suggested Reading

Foley WD, Jochem RJ. Computed tomography: focal and diffuse liver disease. *Radiol Clin North Am* 1991;29:1213.

Part H
PANCREAS

25 Inflammatory Disorders

Acute Pancreatitis

KEY FACTS

- Usually related to alcohol abuse
- Plain radiographs may demonstrate the "colon cutoff" sign, a sentinel loop, gasless abdomen, left-sided pleural effusion, and mottled appearance in the peripancreatic area (fat necrosis)
- Ultrasound findings include:
  a. diffuse or focal enlargement of the pancreas, which appears uniformly hypoechoic (due to inflammatory edema)
  b. areas of increased echogenicity if there is hemorrhage with necrosis, clotted blood, or peripancreatic debris
  c. extrapancreatic hypoechoic mass with good through transmission (phlegmonous pancreatitis)
  d. fluid collection in the lesser sac, anterior and posterior pararenal space
  e. pseudocyst formation
- CT findings include:
  a. diffuse or focal enlargement of the gland
  b. areas of high attenuation in hemorrhagic pancreatitis and low attenuation in phlegmonous pancreatitis
  c. obliteration of the peripancreatic soft tissues and thickening of surrounding fascial planes (extrapancreatic spread of inflammation and edema, especially into the anterior pararenal space, lesser sac, and transverse mesocolon)
  d. after contrast injection, nonenhancing portions of the parenchyma reflect areas of pancreatic necrosis
- Dilatation of the pancreatic duct with proximal dilatation (on ultrasound or CT) may be due to inflammation, spasm, edema, swelling of the papilla, an impacted gallstone, or an associated pseudocyst
- Focal enlargement of the head of the pancreas may be indistinguishable from a neoplasm

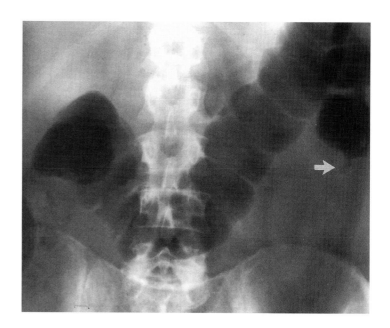

FIGURE 25-1   Acute pancreatitis (colon cutoff sign). The colonic gas column is
abruptly cut off just distal to the splenic flexure *(arrow)*.

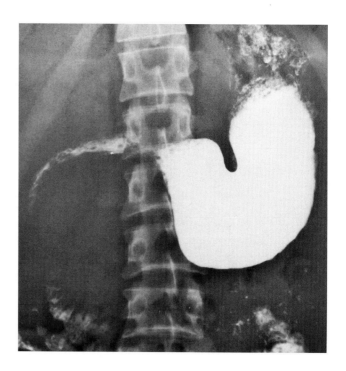

FIGURE 25-2

Acute pancreatitis. Severe
inflammation causes
widening of the sweep and a
high-grade duodenal
obstruction.

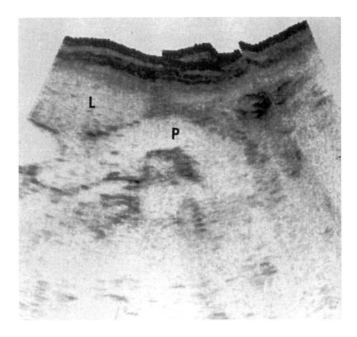

FIGURE 25-3   Acute pancreatitis. Transverse sonogram demonstrates diffuse enlargement of the gland with retention of its normal shape. Note the relative sonolucency of the pancreas *(P)* when compared with the echogenicity of the adjacent liver.

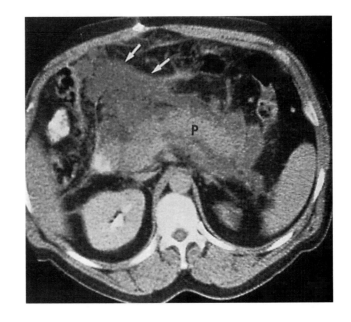

FIGURE 25-4
Acute pancreatitis. CT scan shows diffuse enlargement of the pancreas *(P)*, with obliteration of peripancreatic fat planes by the inflammatory process. Note the extension of the inflammatory reaction into the transverse mesocolon *(arrows)*. (From Jeffrey RB, Federle MD, Laing FC. Computed tomography of mesenteric involvement in fulminant pancreatitis. *Radiology* 1983;147:185, with permission.)

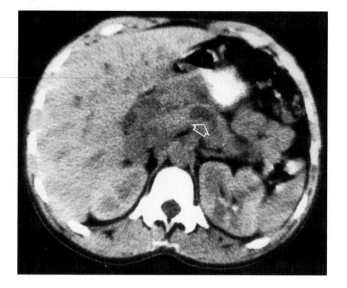

FIGURE 25-5

Acute pancreatitis. CT scan shows generalized enlargement of the head of the pancreas with dilatation of the pancreatic duct *(arrow)*.

Suggested Reading

Balthazar EJ, Robinson DL, Megibow AJ, et al. Acute pancreatitis: value of CT in establishing prognosis. *Radiology* 1990;174:331.

Chronic Pancreatitis

KEY FACTS

- Caused by recurrent and prolonged bouts of acute pancreatitis that lead to pancreatic atrophy and progressive fibrosis
- More than half the patients have a long history of alcohol abuse; about a third have previous biliary disease (usually with gallstones)
- Radiographically visible irregular calcifications are seen in up to 50% of those with alcoholic pancreatitis
- Chronic inflammatory changes in the pancreas can lead to inflammatory strictures of the common bile duct
- Irregular dilatation of the pancreatic duct with strictures and stenoses
- Ultrasound findings include:
  a. gland may be small and atrophic, or diffusely or focally enlarged (often representing edema associated with an acute exacerbation)
  b. heterogeneous gland with areas of increased echogenicity (due to fat and fibrosis)
  c. strong ductal echoes with posterior acoustic shadowing (due to pancreatic calculi)
- CT also can demonstrate ductal dilatation, calcification, and atrophy of the gland
- Endoscopic retrograde cholangiopancreatography (ERCP) may show duct strictures, side branch enlargement, and intraluminal filling defects

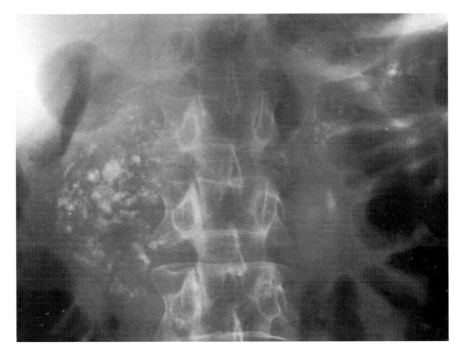

FIGURE 25-6   Chronic pancreatitis. Diffuse pancreatic calcifications.

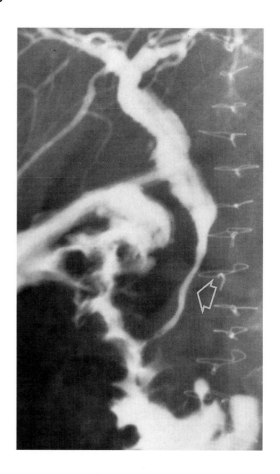

FIGURE 25-7
Chronic pancreatitis. Smooth narrowing of the intrapancreatic portion of the common bile duct *(arrow)*. Note the associated thickening of folds in the adjacent second portion of the duodenum.

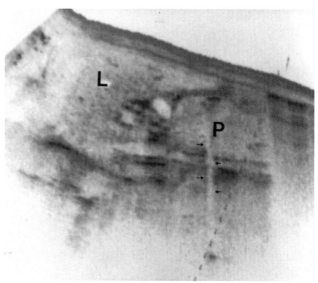

FIGURE 25-8
Chronic pancreatitis. Sonogram shows echogenic pancreas *(P)* containing diffuse calcifications *(arrowheads). L,* liver. (From Krebs CA, Giyanani VL, Eisenberg RL. *Ultrasound atlas of disease processes.* Norwalk, CT: Appleton & Lange, 1993, with permission.)

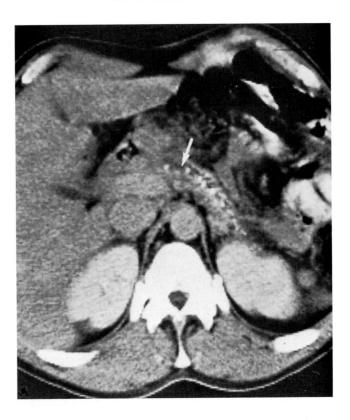

FIGURE 25-9   Chronic pancreatitis. CT scan shows pancreatic atrophy along with multiple intraductal calculi and dilatation of the pancreatic duct *(arrow)*. The calcifications were not seen on plain abdominal radiographs. (From Moss AA, Gamsu G, Genant HK. *Computed tomography of the body.* Philadelphia: WB Saunders, 1983, with permission.)

Suggested Reading
Luetmer PH, Stephens DH, Ward EM. Chronic pancreatitis: reassessment with current CT. *Radiology* 1989;171:353.

Pancreatic Abscess

KEY FACTS

- Serious and often fatal complication of acute pancreatitis
- On plain radiographs, pancreatic fat necrosis produces a pathognomonic mottled pattern of speckled radiolucencies that do not follow the distribution of normal bowel
- On ultrasound, a complex, predominantly cystic mass that often has irregular walls and internal debris
- Bright echoes in the mass (representing gas) confirm the diagnosis of an abscess
- On CT, poorly defined, inhomogeneous mass that often displaces adjacent structures and generally has an attenuation value higher than that of a sterile fluid collection or pseudocyst
- Most reliable sign of an abscess is gas in the mass, though this is found in <50% of cases and may also occur if a pseudocyst erodes into the gastrointestinal tract without abscess formation

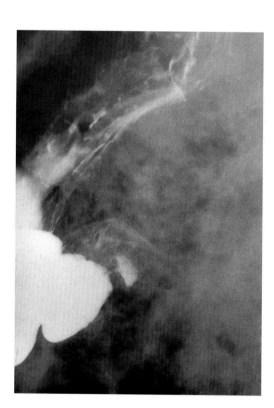

FIGURE 25-10

Pancreatic abscess. Characteristic mottled pattern of speckled radiolucencies, with normal fat intermingled with areas of water density, involves much of the retroperitoneal space.

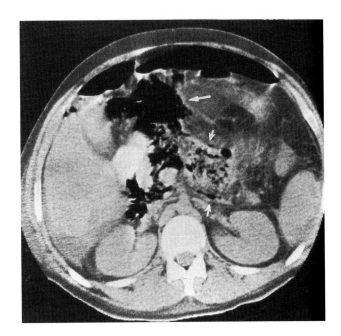

FIGURE 25-11

Pancreatic abscess. There is a gas-containing abscess *(small arrows)* in the pancreatic bed, with marked anterior extension *(large arrow)* of the inflammatory process.

Suggested Reading

Freeny PC. Radiology of the pancreas: two decades of progress in imaging and intervention. *AJR* 1988;150:975.

Pancreatic Pseudocyst

KEY FACTS

- Encapsulated collection of fluid with a high concentration of pancreatic enzymes
- So named because it does not possess the epithelial lining that is characteristic of true cysts
- Arises from inflammation, necrosis, or hemorrhage related to acute pancreatitis or trauma
- About 70% arise from the body and tail of the pancreas; those arising from the head of the gland can widen and compress the duodenal sweep
- Complications include rupture, hemorrhage, and infection
- On ultrasound, uncomplicated pseudocysts are usually anechoic with smooth walls and good sound transmission
- Pseudocysts infrequently are multiloculated, have thick walls, and contain internal debris (difficult to distinguish from cystic pancreatic neoplasms)
- On CT, sharply marginated fluid-filled collection that is often best delineated after contrast administration
- CT may demonstrate pseudocysts that have dissected superiorly into the mediastinum or to other ectopic locations (such as the lumbar or inguinal region or within the liver, spleen or kidney)

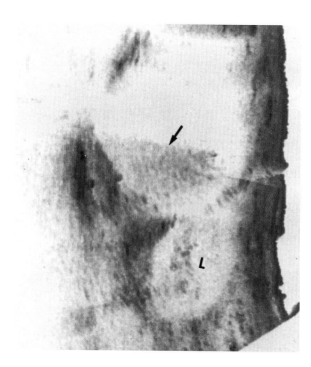

FIGURE 25-12

Pancreatic pseudocyst. Erect sonogram demonstrates a fluid-debris level *(arrow)* in the pseudocyst, situated just above the left kidney *(L)*.

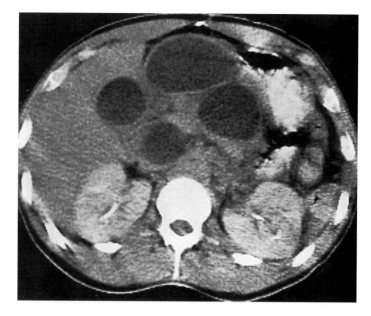

FIGURE 25-13 Multiple pancreatic pseudocysts. CT scan demonstrates four sharply marginated fluid-filled collections.

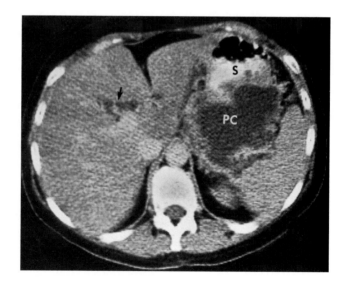

FIGURE 25-14

Ectopic pancreatic pseudocyst. CT scan shows the pseudocyst *(PC)* in the superior recess of the lesser sac, posterior to the stomach *(S)*. Note the dilated intrahepatic bile ducts *(arrow)*.

Suggested Reading

Freeny PC. Radiology of the pancreas: two decades of progress in imaging and intervention. *AJR* 1988;150:975.

26   Neoplasms

Pancreatic Carcinoma

KEY FACTS

- Highly lethal tumor that is usually unresectable at time of presentation
- Increased incidence in patients with history of alcohol abuse, diabetes, smoking, and hereditary pancreatitis
- On barium studies, classic antral pad and Frostberg's "inverted-3" signs, with irregular narrowing and spiculation of the duodenal sweep
- On ultrasound, an irregular, solid hypoechoic mass with low-level echoes and increased sound absorption (infrequently, densely hyperechoic)
- On CT, a mass of decreased attenuation when compared with the normally enhancing pancreas
- Some necrotic tumors have well-defined borders and a uniform low density simulating a pseudocyst
- Smooth or irregular dilatation of the pancreatic duct may occur (as in pancreatitis)
- Carcinoma of the head of the pancreas can encircle and asymmetrically narrow or even obstruct the common bile duct
- Because a focal mass can also be seen in acute or chronic pancreatitis, a diagnosis of carcinoma requires evidence of secondary signs of malignancy such as encasement of adjacent vessels, lymph node enlargement, and liver metastases

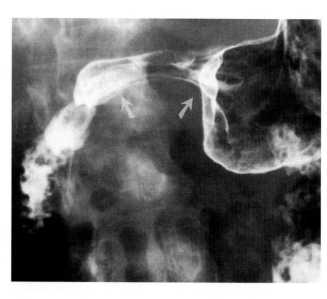

FIGURE 26-1

Pancreatic carcinoma (antral pad sign). Indentation on the greater curvature of the stomach *(arrows)* due to the large pancreatic mass.

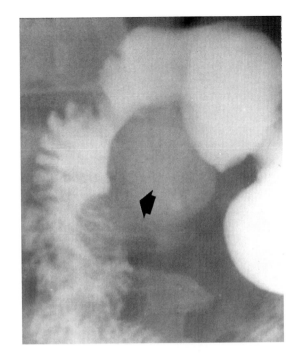

FIGURE 26-2
Pancreatic carcinoma (Frostberg's "inverted-3" sign). The central limb of the 3 *(arrow)* represents the point of fixation of the duodenal wall, where the pancreatic and common bile ducts insert into the papilla.

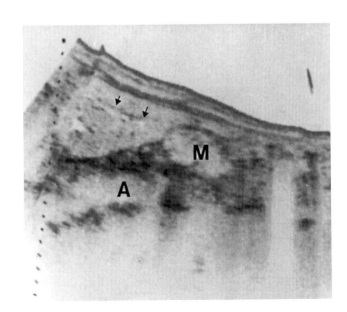

FIGURE 26-3
Pancreatic carcinoma. Longitudinal sonogram demonstrates an irregular mass *(M)* containing a semisolid pattern of intrinsic echoes. There is associated dilatation of the intrahepatic bile ducts *(arrows)*. *A*, aorta.

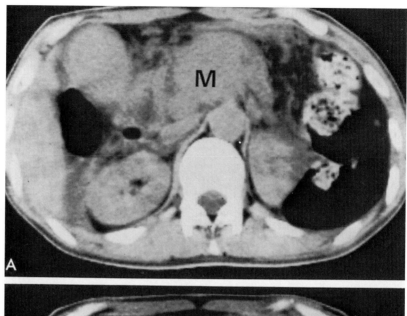

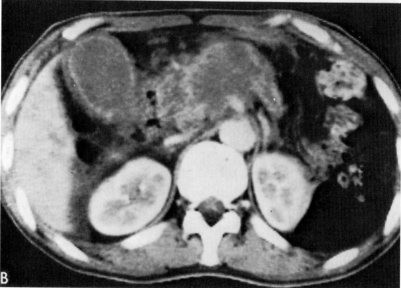

FIGURE 26-4 Pancreatic carcinoma. **A:** Noncontrast CT scan demonstrates a homogeneous mass *(M)* in the body of the pancreas. **B:** Contrast-enhanced scan shows enhancement of the surrounding vascular structures and normal pancreatic parenchyma while the pancreatic carcinoma remains unchanged and thus appears as a low-density mass. (From Federle MP, Goldberg HI. Computed tomography of the pancreas. In: Moss AA, Gamsu G, Genant HK, eds. *Computed tomography of the body.* Philadelphia: WB Saunders, 1983, with permission.)

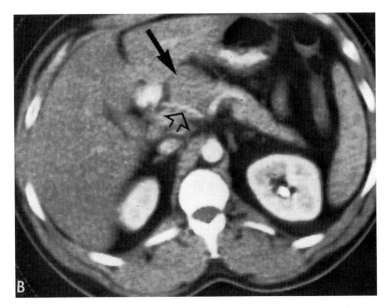

FIGURE 26-5   Pancreatic carcinoma. Dynamic CT scan after the intravenous bolus injection of contrast material demonstrates the tumor *(solid arrow)* with the splenic and hepatic arteries at its base. Note that the hepatic artery *(open arrow)* has an irregular contour. Arteriography showed encasement by this unresectable tumor. (From Federle MP, Goldberg HI. Computed tomography of the pancreas. In: Moss AA, Gamsu G, Genant HK, eds. *Computed tomography of the body.* Philadelphia: WB Saunders, 1983, with permission.)

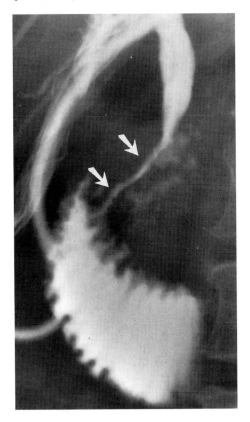

FIGURE 26-6

Pancreatic carcinoma. Irregular narrowing of the common bile duct *(arrows)*. The calcifications reflect underlying chronic pancreatitis.

Suggested Reading

Megibow AJ. Pancreatic adenocarcinoma: designing the examination to evaluate the clinical question. *Radiology* 1992;183:297.

Cystic Pancreatic Neoplasms

MICROCYSTIC ADENOMA (SEROUS CYSTADENOMA)

KEY FACTS

- Benign lobulated neoplasm composed of innumerable small cysts containing proteinaceous fluid and separated by thin connective tissue septa
- About one-third show amorphous central calcifications (sunburst pattern)
- Prominent central stellate fibrotic scar that may calcify is a distinctive feature
- On ultrasound, a solid mass with mixed hypoechoic and echogenic areas
- On CT, a hypodense mass that has a Swiss cheese appearance following contrast administration (due to the numerous tiny cysts)

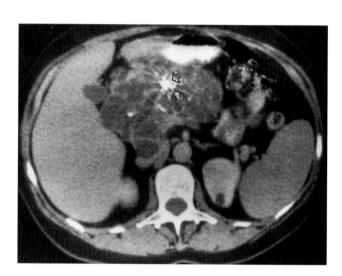

FIGURE 26-7
Microcystic adenoma. CT scan shows a large pancreatic mass with hyperattenuating, enhanced septations and multiple small cystic spaces. Large calcifications are seen in the center of the tumor *(arrows)*.

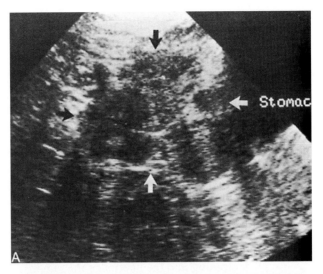

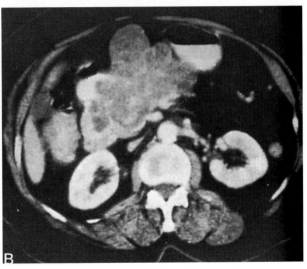

FIGURE 26-8

Microcystic adenoma.
A: Transverse sonogram
demonstrates a solid and
hypoechoic externally
lobulated mass *(arrows)*. The
water-filled stomach is on the
right. **B:** Enhanced CT scan
shows a large lobulated mass
arising from the anterior aspect
of the pancreatic head and
neck. The internal contrast
material enhancement
produces a fine, Swiss cheese
pattern of density and lucency
throughout.

Suggested Reading

Ros PR, Hamrick-Turner JE, Chiechi M, et al. Cystic masses of the pancreas. *Radiographics* 1992;12:673.

MUCINOUS CYSTIC NEOPLASM (CYSTADENOCARCINOMA)

KEY FACTS

- All are either frankly or potentially malignant (metastases to the liver tend to be cystic)
- Composed of large (>5 cm) cystic spaces that are lined with mucin-producing cells and 1- to 2-cm-thick walls
- Most arise in the tail of the pancreas
- Striking female predominance
- On both ultrasound and CT, a predominantly cystic mass with septations and thick irregular walls (may be curvilinear peripheral mural calcifications)
- CT is superior for demonstrating the wall and organ of origin; ultrasound usually is better for showing the septa and any solid excrescences protruding into the interior of the tumor
- Even when malignant, may be potentially curable in the absence of distant metastases

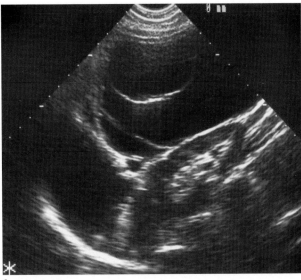

A

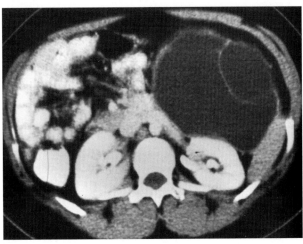

FIGURE 26-9

Mucinous cystic neoplasm. **A:** Sonogram demonstrates a large cystic mass containing septations in the tail of the pancreas. **B:** Contrast-enhanced CT scan reveals a mass with an attenuation coefficient in the range of that of water, with an internal septation and mild nodularity of its wall.

B

Suggested Reading

Ros PR, Hamrick-Turner JE, Chiechi M, et al. Cystic masses of the pancreas. *Radiographics* 1992;12:673.

Pancreatic Islet Cell Tumors

KEY FACTS

- Small hypervascular tumors that are isodense with the normal pancreas on CT and demonstrate characteristic tumor blush on rapid sequential scanning after a bolus injection of contrast
- Larger tumors more commonly demonstrate cystic changes, necrosis, local invasion, vascular invasion, and distant metastases
- Calcifications are rare in functioning tumors
- Often impossible to distinguish these rare tumors from surrounding pancreatic tissue on noncontrast scans

Suggested Reading

Rossi P, Allison DJ, Bezzi M, et al. Endocrine tumors of the pancreas. *Radiol Clin North Am* 1989;27:129.

INSULINOMA

KEY FACTS

- Most common functioning islet cell tumor (arises from beta cells)
- About 90% are single and benign (though multiple adenomas can occur as well as malignant tumors with functional metastases)
- Whipple's triad (symptoms of hypoglycemia; fasting blood glucose ≤40 mg/dL; and immediate resolution of symptoms with intravenous glucose administration)
- Percutaneous venous sampling with insulin assay can localize small or multiple tumors

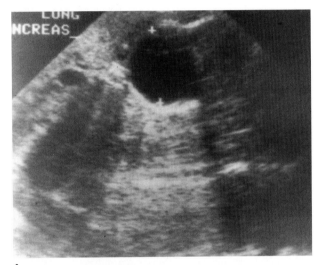

A

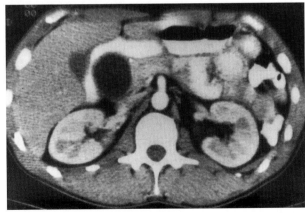

FIGURE 26-10

Insulinoma. **A:** Sonogram demonstrates a cystic mass, with acoustic enhancement and without evidence of debris, in the head of the pancreas. **B:** CT scan shows a cystic mass that displaces the duodenum laterally.

B

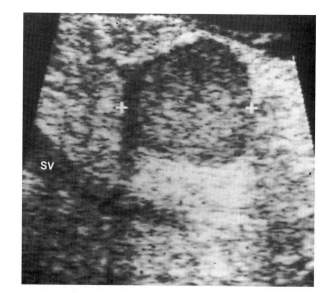

FIGURE 26-11

Insulinoma. Intraoperative
transverse sonogram
demonstrates a hypoechoic
lesion *(cursors)* in the pancreatic
tail. The tubular lucency in the
far field is the splenic vein *(SV)*.

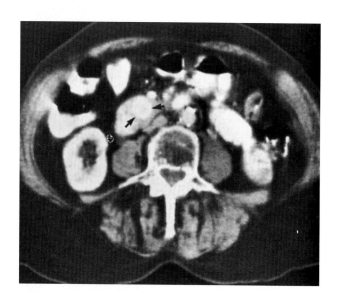

FIGURE 26-12

CT scan shows an enhancing
insulinoma *(arrows)* in the
pancreatic head.

Suggested Reading

Venkatesh S, Ordonez NG, Ajuni J, et al. Islet cell carcinoma of the pancreas. *Cancer* 1990;
    65:354.

GASTRINOMA

KEY FACTS

- Second most common islet cell tumor (arises from alpha/delta cells)
- About 50% are malignant with functioning metastases in regional lymph nodes and liver
- Tumor lies in an ectopic location in about 10% of cases (stomach, duodenum, splenic hilum)
- Association with Zollinger-Ellison syndrome and multiple endocrine neoplasia (MEN)

Suggested Reading
Wank SA, Doppman JL, Miller DL, et al. Prospective study of the ability of computed axial tomography to localize gastrinomas in patients with Zollinger-Ellison syndrome. *Gastroenterology* 1987;92:905.

GLUCAGONOMA

KEY FACTS

- Uncommon tumor derived from alpha cells
- Associated with diabetes, dermatitis, and painful glossitis
- High incidence of malignant transformation (about 80%)

Suggested Reading
Breatnach ES, Hau SY, Rahatzad MT, et al. CT evaluation of glucagonomas. *J Comput Assist Tomogr* 1985;9:25.

VIPOMA

KEY FACTS

- Rare tumor that secretes excessive amount of *v*asoactive *i*ntestinal *p*olypeptide, which causes profuse watery diarrhea with hypokalemia and achlorhydria ("pancreatic cholera")
- High incidence of malignant transformation (about 60%)

Suggested Reading
Mekhjian HS, O'Doriso TJ. Vipoma syndrome. *Semin Oncol* 1987;14:282.

SOMATOSTATINOMA

KEY FACTS

- Rare tumor that suppresses the release of pancreatic and bowel peptides (arises from delta cells)
- Symptoms of diabetes, gallbladder disease, and steatorrhea
- High incidence of malignant transformation (about 90%)

Suggested Reading
Roberts L, Dunnick NR, Foster WL, et al. Somatostatinoma of the endocrine pancreas: CT findings. *J Comput Assist Tomogr* 1984;8:1015.

NONFUNCTIONING ISLET CELL TUMORS

KEY FACTS

- Third most common islet cell tumor (arises from alpha or beta cells)
- Tend to be much larger than functioning tumors and predominantly involve the head of the pancreas
- High incidence of malignant transformation (about 85%)
- Coarse calcifications are relatively common

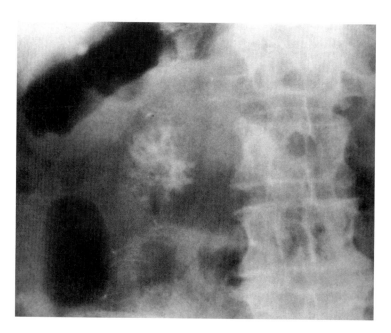

FIGURE 26-13   Pancreatic islet cell tumor (insulinoma). Coarse sunburst calcification in the right upper quadrant.

Suggested Reading

Fugazzola C, Procacci C, Andreis IAB, et al. The contribution of ultrasonography and computed tomography in the diagnosis of nonfunctioning islet cell tumors of the pancreas. *Gastrointest Radiol* 1990;15:139.

SPLEEN

27 Cysts

Splenic Cysts

NONPARASITIC CYSTS

KEY FACTS

- Congenital or secondary to previous infarction or infection
- Solitary, unilocular, homogeneous water-density lesion with pencil-thin margins that do not enhance after contrast administration
- Secondary cysts may demonstrate thin, rim-like calcification

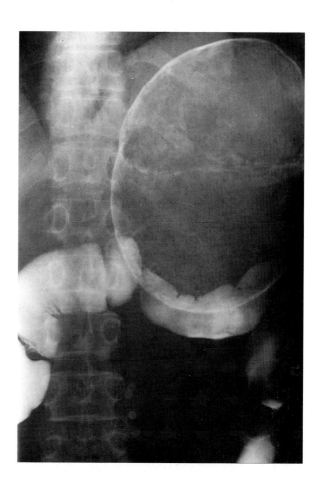

FIGURE 27-1
Huge calcified splenic cyst.

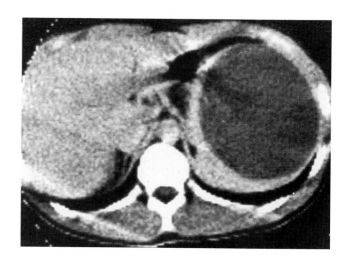

FIGURE 27-2
Congenital cyst. Large, sharply marginated, low-attenuation mass that fills almost all of the spleen. (From Piekarski J, Federle MP, Moss AA, et al. Computed tomography of the spleen. Radiology 1980;135:683, with permission.)

Suggested Reading

Piekarski J, Federle MP, Moss AA, et al. Computed tomography of the spleen. *Radiology* 1980;135:683.

ECHINOCOCCAL (HYDATID) CYST

KEY FACTS

- Spleen is involved in about 2% of cases
- Round or oval mass with sharp margins and near-water density
- Extensive mural calcification that tends to be thick and irregular (unlike the infrequent calcification of congenital cysts, which tends to be thin and smooth)
- Noncalcified portions of the cyst wall enhance with contrast
- Daughter cysts budding from the outer cyst wall often produce a multiloculated appearance

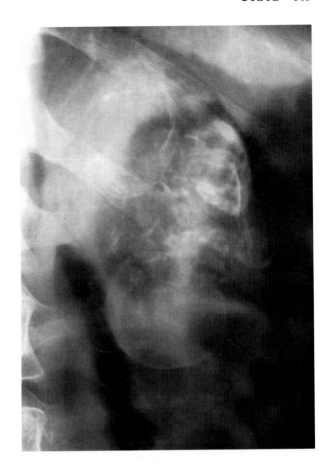

FIGURE 27-3
Echinococcal (hydatid) cyst.
Irregularly calcified mass.

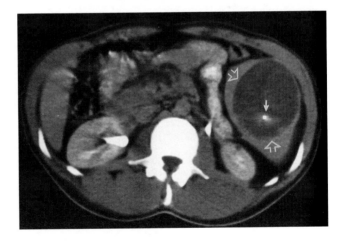

FIGURE 27-4
Echinococcal (hydatid) cyst.
Round, low-attenuation
intrasplenic mass containing
an intracystic calcification
(solid arrow). The cyst has
pencil-sharp margins and an
enhancing rim *(open arrows)*.
(From Piekarski J, Federle
MP, Moss AA, et al.
Computed tomography of the
spleen. *Radiology*
1980;135:683, with
permission.)

Suggested Reading
Franquet T, Montes M, Lecumberri FJ, et al. Hydatid disease of the spleen: imaging findings
   in nine patients. *AJR* 1990;154:525.

28 Abscesses

Splenic Abscess

PYOGENIC ABSCESS

KEY FACTS

- Early diagnosis and prompt treatment are essential to prevent such complications as rupture, subphrenic abscess, and peritonitis
- About 75% are associated with the hematogenous spread of infection, 15% with trauma, and 10% with splenic infarction
- On CT, single or, more commonly, multiple round, low-attenuation masses with ill-defined, thick and irregular walls that usually do not show contrast enhancement
- Though relatively infrequent, the presence of gas within the mass is virtually diagnostic

FIGURE 28-1
Pyogenic abscess. Low-attenuation mass within the spleen *(white arrow)*, with inflammatory soft-tissue stranding in the adjacent extraperitoneal fat *(black arrow)*. There is minimal ascites surrounding the liver. (From Rabushka LS, Kawashima A, Fishman EK: Imaging of the spleen: CT with supplemental MR examination. *Radiographics* 1994;14:307, with permission.)

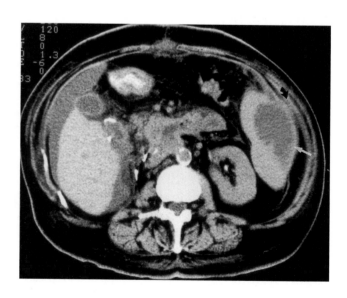

FIGURE 28-2

Pyogenic abscess. Enlarged spleen containing a massive amount of gas. There presence of perisplenic gas and fluid indicates rupture of the spleen *(straight solid arrow)*. The inflammation extends into the adjacent perisplenic fat *(open arrow)*. Note the retroperitoneal gas adjacent to the right adrenal gland *(curved solid arrow)*. (From Rabushka LS, Kawashima A, Fishman EK: Imaging of the spleen: CT with supplemental MR examination. *Radiographics* 1994;14:307, with permission.)

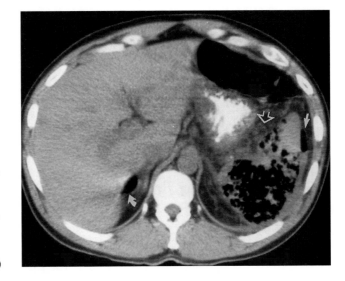

Suggested Reading

Rabushka LS, Kawashima A, Fishman EK. Imaging of the spleen: CT with supplemental MR examination. *Radiographics* 1994;14:307.

FUNGAL MICROABSCESSES

KEY FACTS

- Occur almost exclusively in immunocompromised patients
- On CT, multiple well-defined, nonenhancing low-attenuation lesions
- Occasionally exhibit the characteristic finding of central foci of high-attenuation within the low-attenuation lesions

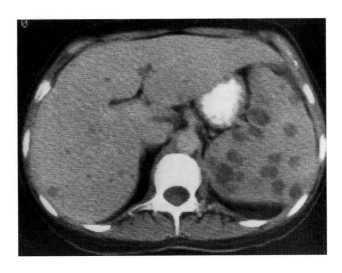

FIGURE 28-3

Fungal abscesses. Multiple low-attenuation lesions within the spleen in an immunocompromised patient.

Suggested Reading

Chew FS, Smith PL, Barboriak D. Candidal splenic abscesses. *AJR* 1991;156:474.

29 Neoplasms

Lymphoma of the Spleen

KEY FACTS

- Most common malignant tumor of the spleen
- The spleen is involved in about 40% of patients at the time of initial presentation and is often the only site of involvement in patients with Hodgkin's disease
- Most common CT appearance is generalized enlargement of a normal-density spleen without evidence of a discrete mass
- Infrequently, lymphoma causes single or multiple focal low-attenuation lesions

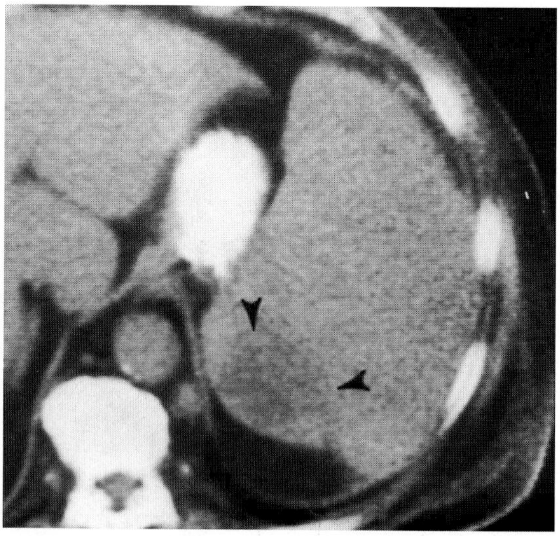

FIGURE 29-1

Lymphoma. Focal low-attenuation lesion *(arrowheads)* located posteriorly in a markedly enlarged spleen. (From Lee JKT, Sagel SS, Stanley RJ. *Computed body tomography.* New York: Raven Press, 1988, with permission.)

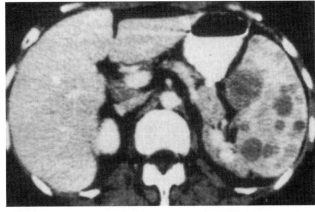

A

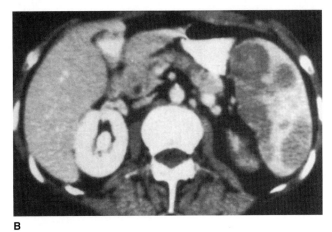

B

FIGURE 29-2
Lymphoma. Multiple discrete low-attenuation lesions in an enlarged spleen. (From Fishman EK, Kuhlman JE, Jones RJ. CT of lymphoma: spectrum of disease. *Radiographics* 1991;11:647, with permission.)

Suggested Reading

Fishman EK, Kuhlman JE, Jones RJ. CT of lymphoma: spectrum of disease. *Radiographics* 1991;11:647.

Metastases to the Spleen

KEY FACTS

- Relatively uncommon site of metastases (primarily hematogenous)
- Most frequently arise from melanoma and primary carcinomas of the breast and lung
- Single or multiple low-attenuation lesions that range from ill-defined hypodense areas to well-delineated cystic masses
- Metastatic nodules with areas of necrosis and liquefaction can contain irregularly shaped regions that approach water density.
- Cyst-like masses may show contrast enhancement of the periphery and septa

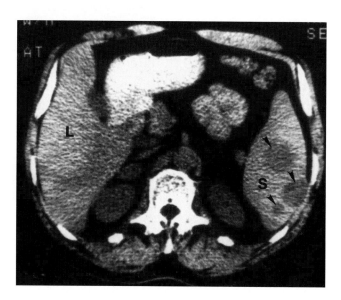

FIGURE 29-3
Metastases to the spleen. Three discrete low-attenuation lesions *(arrowheads)* in the spleen *(S)*. *L*, liver. (From Krebs CA, Giyanani VL, Eisenberg RL. *Ultrasound atlas of disease processes.* Norwalk, CT: Appleton & Lange, 1993, with permission.)

Suggested Reading

Krebs CA, Giyanani VL, Eisenberg RL. *Ultrasound atlas of disease processes.* Norwalk, CT: Appleton & Lange, 1993.

30   Other Disorders

Accessory Spleen

KEY FACTS

- Relatively common failure of mesodermal splenic buds to coalesce into a single organ
- Most common locations are the splenic hilum, gastrohepatic ligament, and other suspensory ligaments of the spleen
- After splenectomy, accessory splenic tissue hypertrophies and can cause recurrence of hematologic disorders (idiopathic thrombocytopenic purpura, hereditary spherocytosis, acquired autoimmune hemolytic anemia, hypersplenism)
- Radionuclide technetium (Tc-99m) sulfur colloid scan demonstrates the splenic tissue (though infrequently identified when the normal spleen is present)

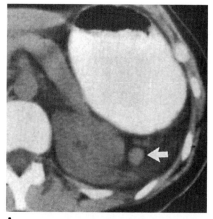

A

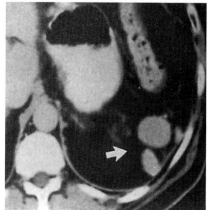

B

FIGURE 30-1

A: Solitary accessory spleen. The smooth mass *(arrow)*, which is located lateral to the kidney, has the same attenuation as the more cephalad main spleen (not shown). **B:** Multiple accessory spleens. On this CT image, three accessory spleens *(arrow)* are seen in the fat of the gastrorenal ligament. Three additional accessory spleens were present at more caudal levels. A main spleen was absent. **C:** Ectopic wandering spleen. Hepatic scintigram (anterior view) obtained to evaluate an incidentally noted asymptomatic, soft midline mass in the mid-abdomen shows a normal-appearing liver in the upper abdomen. The ventral wandering spleen is seen in the midline, just caudal to the liver. There is no normal spleen in the left upper quadrant. (From Dodds WJ, Taylor AJ, Erickson SJ, et al. Radiologic imaging of splenic anomalies. AJR 1990;155:805–810, with permission.)

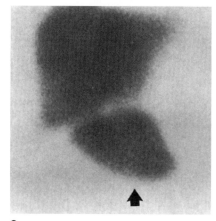

C

Suggested Reading

Dachman AH. The spleen: anomalies and congenital disorders. In: Friedman AC, ed. *Radiology of the liver, biliary tract, pancreas, and spleen.* Baltimore: Williams & Wilkins, 1987.

Splenic Hematoma

KEY FACTS

- The spleen is the intraperitoneal organ that is most frequently injured in blunt abdominal trauma
- Initially, a hematoma may appear isodense or even slightly hyperdense (after contrast injection, may seem to have lower attenuation than the normally enhancing surrounding splenic tissue)
- By 1 to 2 weeks, a gradual decrease in attenuation and nonhomogeneity (decrease in hemoglobin and increased water content) until the hematoma becomes a homogeneous low-attenuation lesion
- *Subcapsular* hematomas appear as crescentic collections of fluid that flatten or indent the lateral margin of the spleen
- *Intrasplenic* hematomas are less common and produce focal masses
- Splenic *lacerations* appear as linear or stellate low-attenuation lesions that do not extend completely across the spleen

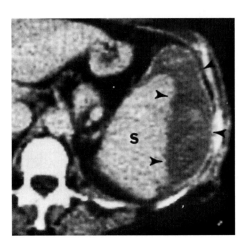

FIGURE 30-2
Subcapsular hematoma. Contrast-enhanced scan shows the hematoma as a large zone of decreased attenuation *(arrowheads)* that surrounds and flattens the lateral and anteromedial borders of the adjacent spleen *(S)*. (From Lee JKT, Sagel SS, Stanley RJ. *Computed body tomography.* New York: Raven Press, 1988, with permission.)

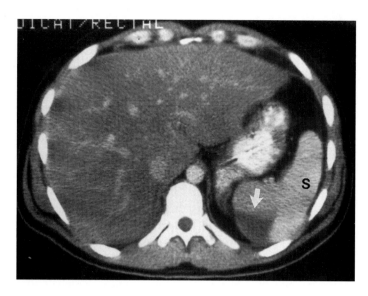

FIGURE 30-3   Splenic laceration. Linear low-attenuation lesions *(arrows)* in the spleen *(S)*. Note the associated subcapsular hematoma. (From Gay SB, Sistrom CL. Computed tomographic evaluation of blunt abdominal trauma. *Radiol Clin North Am* 1992;30:375, with permission.)

Suggested Reading

Gay SB, Sistrom CL. Computed tomography of blunt abdominal trauma. *Radiol Clin North Am* 1992;30:375.

Splenic Infarction

KEY FACTS

- Most commonly results from embolic phenomena or local thrombosis due to hematologic disease

- Classic wedge-shaped area of decreased attenuation that extends to the capsule of the spleen and does not show contrast enhancement (seen in only one-third of cases)

- May present as a heterogeneous, poorly marginated or mass-like low-attenuation region that is indistinguishable from other splenic lesions

- Chronic infarctions show progressive volume loss due to fibrous contraction of the infarct with hypertrophy of the surrounding normal spleen

- In sickle cell disease, chronic infarction can result in a small, densely calcified spleen (autosplenectomy)

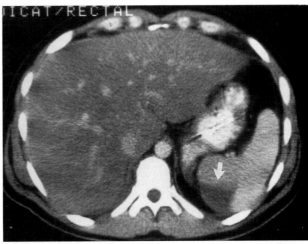

FIGURE 30-4
Infarction. Wedge-shaped, low-attenuation lesion *(arrow)* in the periphery of the spleen. *S,* stomach. (From Krebs CA, Giyanani VL, Eisenberg RL. *Ultrasound atlas of disease processes.* Norwalk, CT: Appleton & Lange, 1993, with permission.)

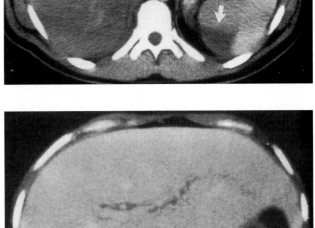

FIGURE 30-5
Autosplenectomy in sickle cell disease. Small, densely calcified spleen. (From Moss AA, Gamsu G, Genant HK, eds. *Computed tomography of the body with magnetic resonance imaging.* Philadelphia: WB Saunders, 1992, with permission.)

Suggested Reading
Balcar I, Seltzer SE, Davis S, et al. CT patterns of splenic infarction: a clinical and experimental study. *Radiology* 1984;151:723.

Splenosis

KEY FACTS

- Autotransplantation of splenic tissue to other sites following trauma
- Major locations include the diaphragmatic surface, liver, omentum, mesentery, peritoneum, and pleura
- Multiple small encapsulated sessile implants
- Most sensitive radionuclide study to show isotope uptake within the ectopic spleen utilizes Tc-99m heat-damaged red blood cells (RBCs) (sulfur colloid or In-labeled platelets also can be employed)

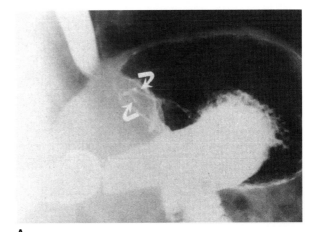

A

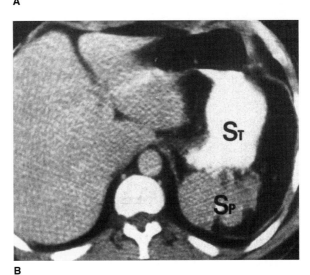

B

FIGURE 30-6
Regenerated splenosis. **A:** Distortion of the gastric fundus by a mass lesion, with overlying linear ulceration *(arrows)*. The sharp margins of the mass suggest an intramural, extramucosal location. **B:** CT scan at the level of the fundus shows a lobulated, homogeneous mass indenting the gastric fundus from behind and medially. Note the absence of the spleen because of a previous splenectomy. *ST*, stomach; *SP*, regenerated spleen. **C:** Radionuclide liver-spleen scan confirms that the mass indenting the gastric fundus indeed represents splenic tissue. *LL*, left lateral; *POS*, posterior. (From Agha FP. Regenerated splenosis masquerading as gastric fundic mass. *Am J Gastroenterol* 1984;79:576, with permission.)

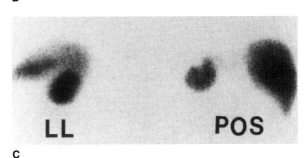

C

Suggested Reading

Agha FP. Regenerated splenosis masquerading as gastric fundal mass. *Am J Gastroenterol* 1984;79:576.

Part J

APPENDIX, MESENTERY, PERITONEAL CAVITY

31   Appendix

Appendicitis

- Produced by a fecalith or postinflammatory scarring that occludes the neck of the appendix and creates a closed-loop obstruction within the organ
- Resulting stasis leads to bacterial infection, thinning and ulceration of the wall, and eventually perforation resulting in the development of a localized abscess or generalized peritonitis
- On barium studies, classically an irregular impression at the base of the cecum (inflammatory edema) associated with failure of barium to enter the appendix
- Calcified appendicoliths which can be demonstrated on plain films in 10% to 15% of cases of acute appendicitis (30% on CT), suggest that the appendix is likely to perforate, and can sometimes be found in ectopic locations (pelvis, right upper quadrant)
- On ultrasound, the inflamed appendix appears as a noncompressible, thick-walled, fluid-filled tubular structure
- On transverse sections, the inflamed appendix has a diameter >6 mm and often has a target configuration
- Appendiceal abscess appears as a complex hypoechoic mass adjacent to the cecum or appendix
- On CT, the inflamed wall of the appendix is homogeneously thickened and shows contrast enhancement
- A critical finding is linear stranding and haziness of the mesenteric fat (representing periappendiceal inflammation)
- Phlegmons appear as pericecal soft-tissue masses; abscesses are seen as pericecal fluid collections (may appear solid if they contain high-density pus and necrotic tissue)

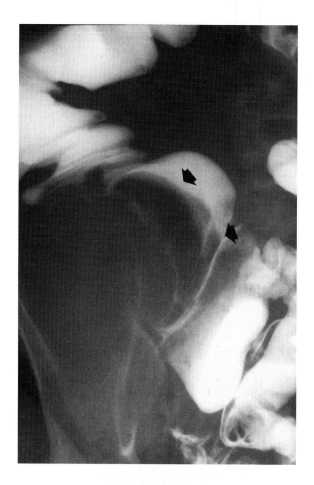

FIGURE 31-1

Appendicitis (periappendiceal abscess). Large extrinsic mass involving the lateral aspect of the ascending colon *(arrows)* secondary to rupture of a retrocecal appendix).

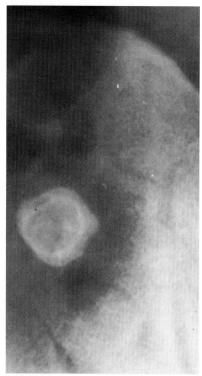

FIGURE 31-2

Appendicolith. Laminated pattern of calcification in the right lower quadrant.

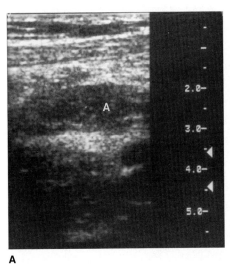

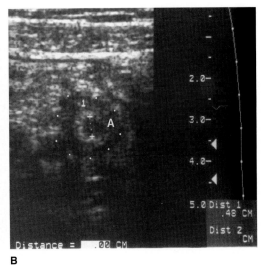

A   **B**

F I G U R E   3 1 - 3   Appendicitis. **A:** Sagittal sonogram shows that the inflamed appendix *(A)* is elongated and hypoechoic and has a central sonolucent lumen *(arrowhead)*. **B:** Transverse scan shows that the inflamed appendix *(A)* has a sonolucent lumen *(cursors)* surrounded by hypoechoic inflamed tissue *(dots)*. (From Krebs CA, Giyanani VL, Eisenberg RL. *Ultrasound atlas of disease processes.* Norwalk, CT: Appleton & Lange, 1993, with permission.)

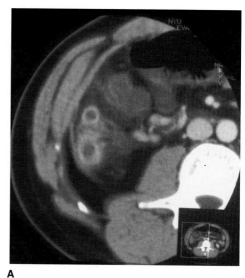

A

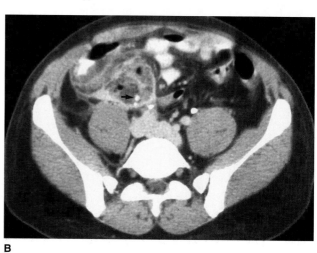

B

FIGURE 31-4

Appendicitis. **A:** On this CT scan, the inflamed U-shaped appendix appears as two dilated, thick-walled tubular structures. Note the pericecal inflammatory changes. **B:** In another patient, there is an appendicolith *(arrow)* within a large appendiceal abscess. (Courtesy of Emil J. Balthazar, M.D.)

Suggested Reading

Balthazar EJ, Megibow AJ, Hulnick D, et al. CT of appendicitis. *AJR* 1986;147:705.

Mucocele of the Appendix

KEY FACTS

- Cystic dilatation of the appendix resulting from proximal luminal obstruction (caused by a fecalith, foreign body, tumor, adhesions, or volvulus), which leads to the accumulation of sterile mucus distally
- Globular, smooth-walled, broad-based mass indenting the lower part of the cecum (usually on the medial side and with no filling of the appendix)
- May have mottled or rim-like calcification around the periphery
- On CT, a sharply defined mass with homogeneous low attenuation
- Rupture of an appendiceal (or ovarian) mucocele can lead to the development of pseudomyxoma peritonei

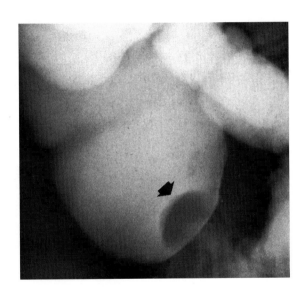

FIGURE 31-5

Muocele of the appendix. Smooth, broad-based filling defect *(arrow)* indenting the lower part of the cecum. The appendix does not fill with barium.

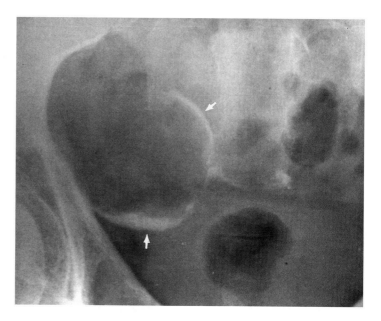

F I G U R E   3 1 - 6   Mucocele of the appendix. Large cystic mass with an incomplete rim of calcification *(arrows)*. (From Baker SR, Elkin M. *Plain film approach to abdominal calcifications.* Philadelphia: WB Saunders, 1983, with permission.)

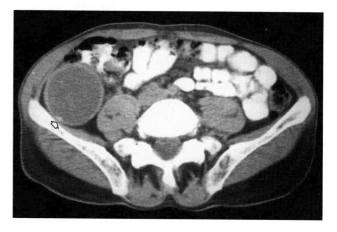

F I G U R E   3 1 - 7   Mucocele of the appendix. CT scan shows a homogeneous low-attenuation mass in the right lower quadrant with anteromedial displacement of the adjacent cecum. Note the high-attenuation area *(arrow)* within the wall posteriorly, representing a fleck of calcification. (From Horgan JG, Chow PP, Richter JO, et al. CT and sonography in the recognition of mucocele of the appendix. *AJR* 1984;143:959, with permission.)

Suggested Reading

Horgan JG, Chow PP, Richter JO, et al. CT and sonography in the recognition of mucocele of the appendix. *AJR* 1984;143:959.

Myxoglobulosis of the Appendix

KEY FACTS

- Rare type of mucocele composed of multiple round or oval translucent globules mixed with mucus
- Usually asymptomatic
- Radiographically indistinguishable from simple mucocele on barium studies
- Characteristic appearance of calcified rim about the periphery of individual globules

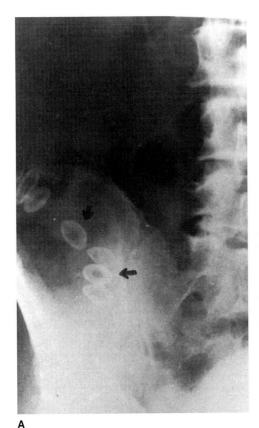 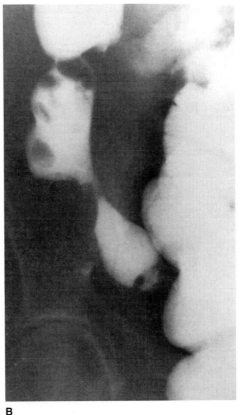

A   B

FIGURE 31-8   Myxoglobulosis of the appendix. **A:** Multiple annular and ovoid spheres of calcification *(arrows)* in the right lower quadrant of the abdomen. **B:** Barium enema shows a huge sac extending down from a contract cecum and containing partially translucent ovid bodies with thick calcified rims. (From Alcalay J, Alkalay L, Lorent T. Myxoglobulosis of the appendix. *Br J Radiol* 1985;58:183, with permission.)

Suggested Reading
Alcalay J, Alkalay L, Lorent T. Myxoglobulosis of the appendix. *Br J Radiol* 1985;58:183.

32 Mesentery

Retractile Mesenteritis

KEY FACTS

- Fibrofatty thickening and sclerosis of the mesentery (probably represents a slowly progressive mesenteric inflammatory process)
- Radiographically appears as a diffuse mesenteric mass that displaces small bowel loops
- If there is prominent fibrosis, the bowel tends to be drawn into a central mass with kinking, angulation, and conglomeration of adherent loops
- On CT, a localized fat-density mass containing areas of increased attenuation representing fibrosis

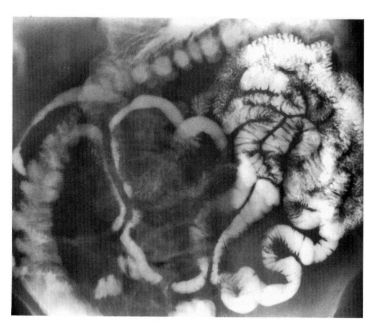

FIGURE 32-1   Retractile mesenteritis. Separation of small bowel folds, which remained constant on successive studies. (From Clement AR, Tracht DG. The roentgen diagnosis of retractile mesenteritis. *AJR* 1969;107:787, with permission.)

FIGURE 32-2
Retractile mesenteritis.
CT scan shows a poorly
defined but fairly localized
fat-density mass within the
right lower quadrant. Multiple
small areas of increased
density within the mass *(white
arrowheads)* represent
enhancement of neurovascular
bundles. Both ureters are well
opacified *(black arrows)*.
(From Seigel RS, Kuhns LR,
Borlaza GS, et al. Computed
tomography and angiography
in ileal carcinoid tumor and
retractile mesenteritis.
Radiology 1980;134:437, with
permission.)

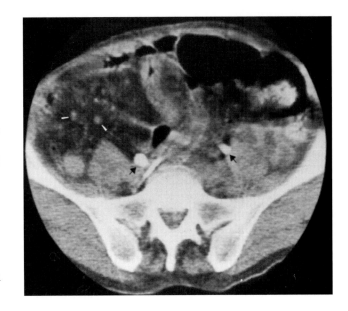

Suggested Reading
Clemett AR, Tracht DG. The roentgen diagnosis of retractile mesenteritis. *AJR* 1969;107:787.

33   Peritoneal Cavity

Ascites

KEY FACTS

- Accumulation of fluid in the peritoneal cavity
- In almost 75% of patients with ascites in the United States, the underlying disease is hepatic cirrhosis (elevated portal venous pressure and decreased serum albumin level)
- Other causes include peritonitis, congestive heart failure, constrictive pericarditis, peritoneal carcinomatosis, and primary or metastatic disease of the lymphatic system
- In the supine patient, ascites tends to collect:
  a. around the inferior tip of the right lobe of the liver
  b. in the superior right flank
  c. in the cul-de-sac
  d. in the paracolic gutters
- Plain radiographs show large amounts of ascites as a general abdominal haziness (ground-glass appearance) with fluid accumulation within the pelvic peritoneal recesses (dog's ears) on supine films
- On ultrasound, mobile echo-free fluid regions shaped by adjacent structures
- On CT, an extravisceral collection of fluid with an attenuation value less than that of adjacent soft-tissue organs

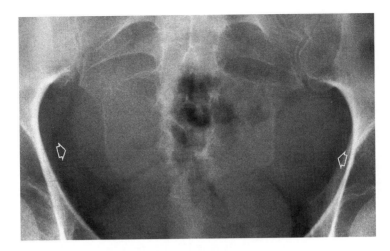

FIGURE 33-1   Ascites. Supine abdominal radiograph demonstrates a large amount of ascitic fluid within the pelvic peritoneal reflections *(arrows)*.

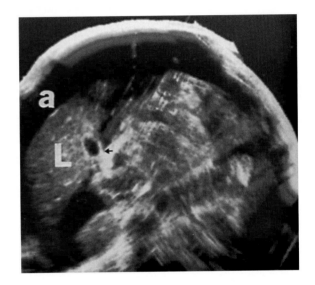

FIGURE 33-2

Ascites. Ultrasound demonstrates a large amount of sonolucent ascitic fluid *(a)* separating the liver *(L)* and other soft-tissue structures from the anterior abdominal wall. Note the relative thickness of the gallbladder wall *(arrow)*.

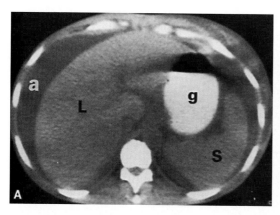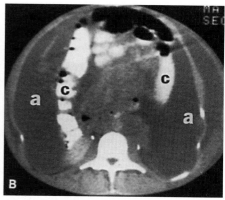

FIGURE 33-3   Ascites. **A:** CT scan through the upper abdomen shows the low-density ascitic fluid *(a)* lateral to the liver *(L)* and spleen *(S)* and separating these structures from the abdominal wall. *G,* barium in the stomach. **B:** Scan through the lower abdomen shows a huge amount of low-density ascitic fluid *(a)* with medial displacement of the ascending and descending colon *(c)*.

Suggested Reading

Krebs CA, Giyanani VL, Eisenberg RL. *Ultrasound atlas of disease processes.* Norwalk, CT: Appleton & Lange, 1993.

Pneumoperitoneum

KEY FACTS

- Major causes of pneumoperitoneum *with* peritonitis include:
  a. perforated viscus
      i. gastric or duodenal ulcer
      ii. colon (toxic megacolon; obstructing malignancy)
  b. penetrating trauma
  c. ulcerative bowel disease (tuberculosis; typhoid fever; Meckel's diverticulum in children)
- Major causes of pneumoperitoneum *without* peritonitis include:
  a. abdominal surgery (usually clears by 3 to 7 days)
  b. rare manifestation of abdominal, gynecologic, or intrathoracic conditions
- Radiographic demonstration of free intraperitoneal gas:
  a. upright projection
  b. double-wall sign or visualization of falciform or other ligaments on supine projection
  c. gas-fluid level over the liver on a decubitus projection with the patient's left side down and using a horizontal x-ray beam
  d. football sign in children (excessive radiolucency of the entire abdomen that often assumes an oval configuration)

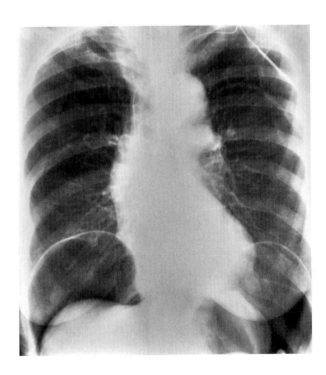

FIGURE 33-4

Pneumoperitoneum. Massive amount of free intraperitoneal gas secondary to perforated viscus.

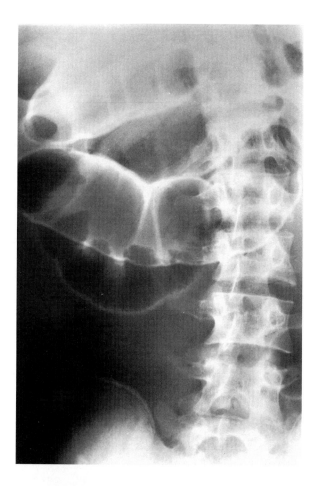

FIGURE 33-5

Pneumoperitoneum (double-wall sign). On this supine view, free intraperitoneal gas may be diagnosed indirectly because the gas permits visualization of the outer margins of the intestinal wall.

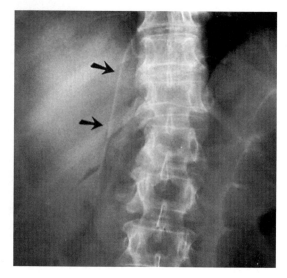

FIGURE 33-6

Pneumoperitoneum (falciform ligament sign). On the supine view, the falciform ligament appears as a curvilinear water density shadow surrounded by free intraperitoneal gas.

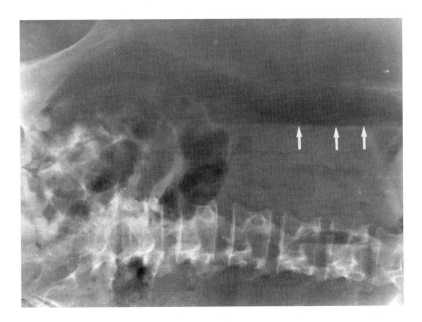

FIGURE 33-7 Pneumoperitoneum. Left lateral decubitus view shows free intraperitoneal gas collecting under the right side of the abdominal wall *(arrows)*. Gas can even be seen extending down the flank to the region of the pelvis. The semierect frontal chest film (not shown) failed to demonstrate any evidence of intraperitoneal gas.

Suggested Reading

Earls JP, Dachman AH, Colon E, et al. Prevalence and duration of postoperative pneumoperitoneum: sensitivity of CT vs left lateral decubitus radiography. *AJR* 1993;161:781.

Peritoneal Metastases

KEY FACTS

- Intraperitoneal seeding results from tumor cells floating freely in ascitic fluid and implanting themselves on peritoneal surfaces
- Typically occurs in the terminal stages of cancer of the intraperitoneal organs (especially ovary and stomach)
- Major areas of involvement include:
  a. pouch of Douglas at the rectosigmoid junction (Blumer's shelf)
  b. right lower quadrant at the lower end of the small bowel mesentery
  c. left lower quadrant along the superior border of the sigmoid mesocolon
  d. right paracolic gutter lateral to the cecum and ascending colon
- CT findings include:
  a. omental cakes (thickening of the greater omentum)
  b. lobulated mass in the pouch of Douglas
  c. adnexal mass of cystic or soft-tissue density (Krukenberg tumor)
  d. loculated fluid collections in the peritoneal cavity
  e. apparent thickening of mesenteric vessels (fluid within leaves of the mesentery)

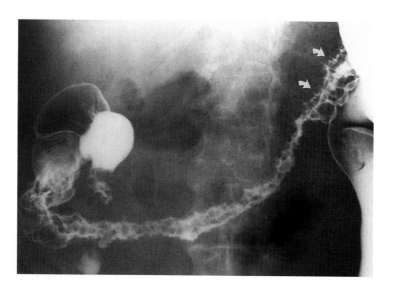

FIGURE 33-8   Peritoneal metastases (omental cakes). Diffuse narrowing and fixation of the transverse colon with severely distorted mucosal folds mimics the cobblestone appearance of Crohn's colitis. There is asymmetric involvement distally with a mass effect and tethered folds on the superior haustral borders *(arrows)*. These findings are the result of diffuse encasement of the transverse colon by omental metastases from bladder carcinoma. (From Rubesin SE, Levine MS. Omental cakes: colonic involvement by omental metastases. *Radiology* 1985;154:593, with permission.)

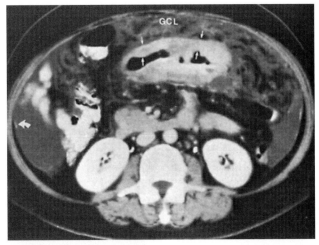

A

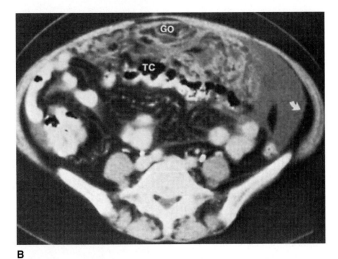

FIGURE 33-9

Peritoneal metastases.
A,B: CT scans show carcinomatous mural thickening of the gastric antrum *(small straight arrows)*. Tumor spread to the gastrocolic ligament *(GCL)* extends into the greater omentum *(GO)*. *Curved arrows*, peritoneal implants; *TC*, transverse colon.
C: Pelvic scan shows bilateral Krukenberg tumors of the ovaries *(solid arrows)*. The appendices epiploicae of the sigmoid mesocolon *(open arrows)* are well demonstrated by the surrounding ascitic fluid. (From Gore RM, Levine MS, Laufer I, eds. *Textbook of gastrointestinal radiology.* Philadelphia: WB Saunders, 1994, with permisssion.)

B

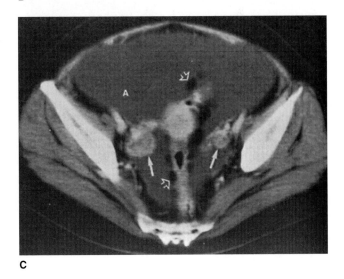

C

Suggested Reading

Gore RM, Levine MS, Laufer I, eds. *Textbook of gastrointestinal radiology.* Philadelphia: WB Saunders, 1994.

Pseudomyxoma Peritonei

KEY FACTS

- Accumulation of large amounts of gelatinous material in the peritoneal cavity
- Caused by rupture of a pseudomucinous cystadenoma of the ovary or mucocele of the appendix
- Widespread annular abdominal calcifications that tend to be most numerous in the pelvis
- Thickening of peritoneal and omental surfaces and scalloping of the liver contour due to diffuse peritoneal implants
- On CT, massive accumulation of low-attenuation gelatinous ascites

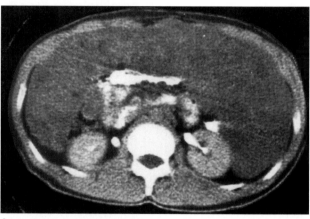

FIGURE 33-10
Pseudomyxoma peritonei.
A: CT scan of the abdomen after rupture of a mucocele of the appendix demonstrates diffuse epithelial implants and gelatinous ascites filling the abdomen. Note the posterior displacement of contrast-filled bowel.
B: Calcification *(arrows)* of serosal implants of pseudomyxoma. (**A**, from Seshul MB, Coulam CM. Pseudomyxoma peritonei: computed tomography and sonography. *AJR* 1981;136:803; **B**, from Madwed D, Mindelzun R, Jeffrey BR. Mucocele of the appendix: imaging findings. *AJR* 1992;159:69, with permission.)

A

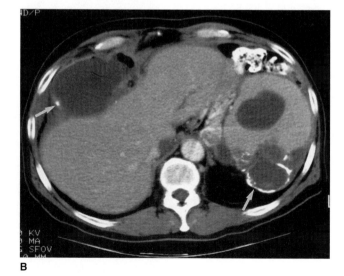

B

Suggested Reading

Seshul MB, Coulam CM. Pseudomyxoma peritonei: computed tomography and sonography. *AJR* 1981;138:803.

MISCELLANEOUS

34   **Miscellaneous Disorders**

Mesenteric Ischemia

KEY FACTS

- Usually a complication of atherosclerosis and cardiac failure in older persons
- Broad spectrum of clinical appearances depending on the rapidity of onset, the length of intestine involved, and the extent of collateral circulation
  - a. rapid occlusion of a major vessel—massive bowel necrosis and death from peritonitis and shock
  - b. insidious onset of segmental involvement—variable amount of damage and healing
- Radiographic findings include:
  - a. regular thickening of small bowel folds (picket fencing)
  - b. thumbprinting in the colon
  - c. separation of bowel loops (bleeding into the mesentery)
  - d. narrowing of the bowel lumen (fibrotic healing)
- Gas in the bowel wall and portal vein is an ominous sign of intestinal infarction

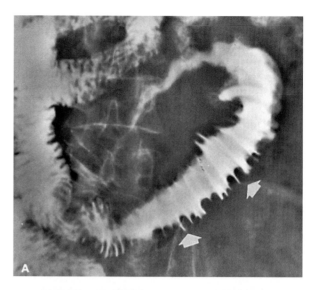

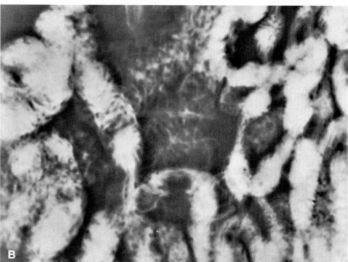

FIGURE 34-1   Mesenteric ischemia. **A:** Segmental ischemia produces a picket-fence pattern of regular thickening of small bowel folds *(arrows)*.
B: Complete resolution of the ischemic process after conservative therapy.

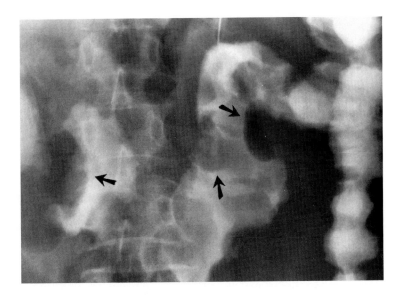

F I G U R E   3 4 - 2   Ischemic colitis. Multiple filling defects *(arrows)* indenting the
margins of the transverse and descending portions of the colon.

Suggested Reading
Lund EC, Han SY, Holleg HC, et al. Intestinal ischemia: comparison of plain radiographic and
computed tomographic findings. *Radiographics* 1988;8:1083.

Necrotizing Enterocolitis

KEY FACTS

- Life-threatening ischemic bowel disease that is secondary to hypoxia, perinatal stress, or infection
- Most common gastrointestinal emergency in premature infants (typically develops within the first 2 weeks of life)
- Primarily involves the ileum and right colon
- Radiographic findings include:
  a. persistently dilated bowel loop or an unchanging bowel gas pattern
  b. frothy or bubbly appearance that suggests feces (but premature infant rarely has stool seen in the colon during the first 2 weeks of life)
- Gas in the bowel wall and portal vein is an ominous sign (though portal vein gas may be transient or related to an umbilical vein catheter)
- On ultrasound, intrahepatic portal vein gas appears as bright reflectors bubbling through the liver
- Late fibrotic strictures may cause clinical and radiographic signs of bowel obstruction

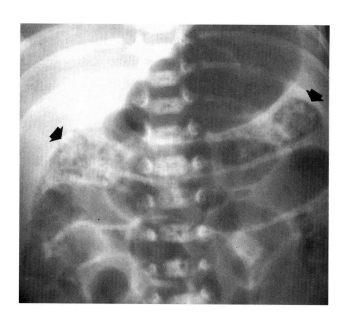

FIGURE 34-3
Necrotizing enterocolitis. Bubbly appearance of gas in the wall of diseased colon of this premature infant resembles fecal material *(arrows)*; although this appearance is normal in adults, it is always abnormal in premature infants.

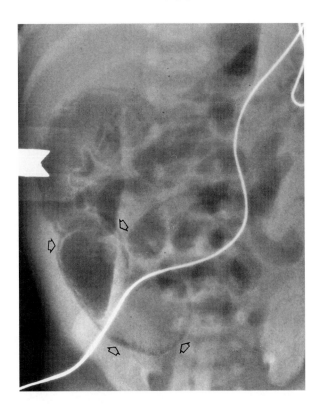

FIGURE 34-4
Necrotizing enterocolitis.
Intramural gas *(arrows)* parallels
the course of the bowel loops.

Suggested Reading

Kogutt MS. Necrotizing enterocolitis of infancy: early roentgen patterns as a guide to prompt diagnosis. *Radiology* 1979;130:367.

Pneumatosis Intestinalis (Gas in the Bowel Wall)

PRIMARY (IDIOPATHIC)

KEY FACTS

- Benign condition with multiple thin-walled, noncommunicating, gas-filled cysts in the bowel wall
- Primarily involves the lower colon
- Asymptomatic with no associated gastrointestinal or respiratory abnormalities (may cause painless pneumoperitoneum)
- Radiolucent clusters of cysts along the contours of the bowel that are compressible on palpation and can simulate polyps, thumbprinting, or even an annular constriction

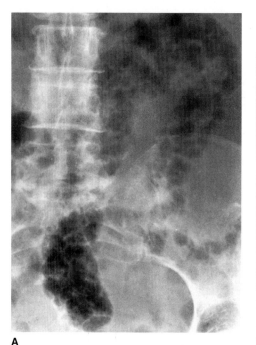 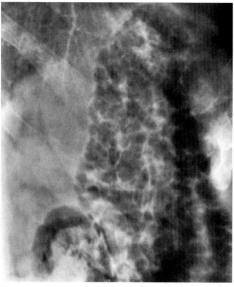

A **B**

FIGURE 34-5 Primary (idiopathic) pneumatosis intestinalis. Radiolucent clusters of gas-filled cysts are seen along the contours of the bowel in the rectosigmoid (**A**) and the splenic flexure (**B**) of this asymptomatic man.

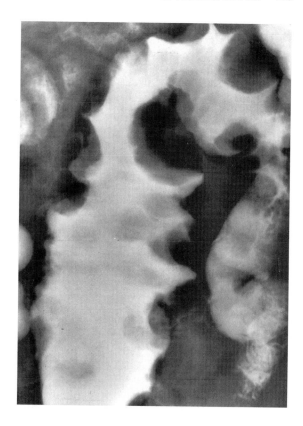

FIGURE 34-6

Primary (idiopathic) pneumatosis intestinalis. In this asymptomatic elderly man, large gas-filled cysts produce scalloped defects in the colon, simulating inflammatory pseudopolyps, thumbprinting, or even multiple neoplasms.

Suggested Reading

Olmsted WW, Madewell JE. Pneumatosis cystoides intestinalis: a pathophysiologic explanation of the roentgenographic signs. *Gastrointest Radiol* 1976;1:177.

SECONDARY

KEY FACTS

- More commonly involves the small bowel, generally has a linear distribution, and is associated with a wide variety of preexisting disorders
- In mesenteric vascular disease, reflects loss of mucosal integrity or increased intraluminal pressure in the bowel (ischemic necrosis; intestinal obstruction, especially if there is strangulation; corrosive ingestion; primary infection of the bowel wall)
- In necrotizing enterocolitis, frothy or bubbly appearance of gas in the wall of diseased bowel may mimic fecal material in the right colon (normal in adults, but abnormal in premature infants)
- Occasionally, gas in the bowel wall reflects gastrointestinal tract disease without necrosis of the bowel wall or obstructive pulmonary disease

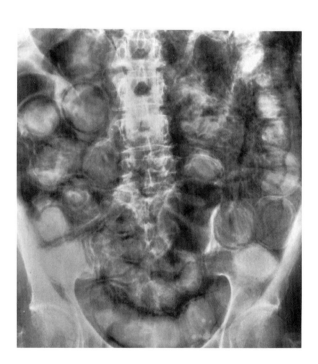

FIGURE 34-7
Secondary pneumatosis intestinalis. Curvilinear gas collections surround virtually all visible bowel loops.

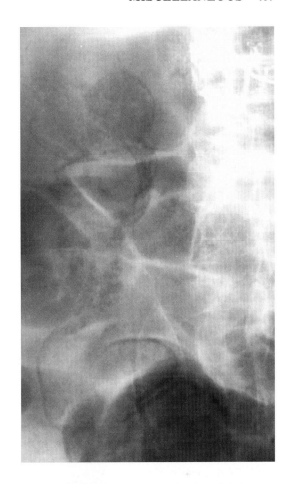

FIGURE 34-8
Secondary pneumatosis intestinalis.
Crescentic linear collections are seen in
the wall of ischemic bowel loops.

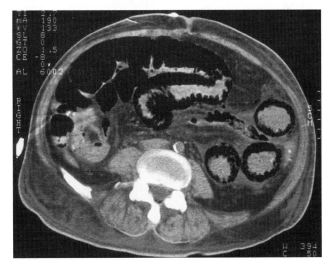

FIGURE 34-9
Secondary pneumatosis
intestinalis. CT scan shows
gas in the bowel wall, which
resolved spontaneously.
(From Feczko PJ, Mezwa
DG, Farah MC, et al. Clinical
significance of pneumatosis
of the bowel wall.
Radiographics 1992;12:1069,
with permission.)

Suggested Reading

Feczko PJ, Mezwa DG, Farah MC, et al. Clinical significance of pneumatosis of the bowel
wall. *Radiographics* 1992;12:1069.

Fistulas

KEY FACTS

- Abnormal communications between the gastrointestinal tract and:
  a. another segment of bowel (enteric-enteric)
  b. another intra-abdominal organ (internal fistula)
  c. the skin (external fistula)
- Major causes of fistulas include Crohn's disease, diverticulitis, malignant neoplasms, radiation therapy, and infectious disorders
- Contrast studies often can demonstrate filling of the fistulous tract

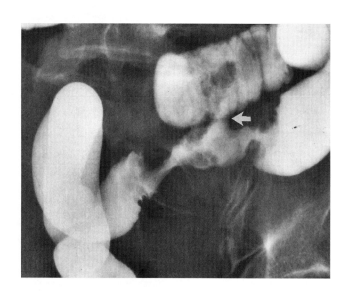

FIGURE 34-10
Malignant ileocolic fistula *(arrow)*. Carcinoma of the sigmoid colon.

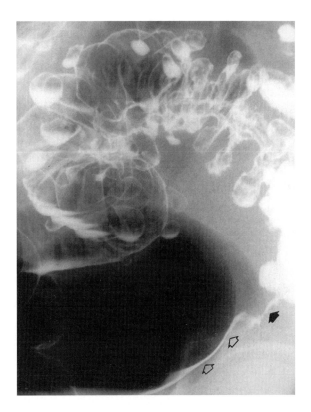

FIGURE 34-11

Colovesical fistula (diverticulitis). Barium enema demonstrates a fistulous tract *(solid arrow)* between the sigmoid colon and the bladder. Barium can also be seen lining the base of the gas-filled bladder *(open arrows)*.

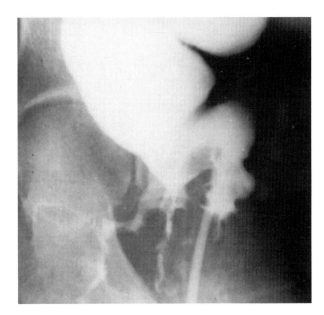

FIGURE 34-12

Perianal fistulas (Crohn's colitis). (From Butch RJ. Radiology of the rectum. In: Taveras JM, Ferrucci JT, eds. *Radiology: diagnosis-imaging-intervention.* Philadelphia: JB Lippincott Co, 1987, with permission.)

Suggested Reading

Eisenberg RL. *Gastrointestinal radiology: a pattern approach.* Philadelphia: Lippincott–Raven Publishers, 1996.

Cystic Fibrosis

KEY FACTS

- Radiographic findings include:
  a. thickened, coarse fold pattern in the first and second portions of the duodenum
  b. adherent fecalith (persistent tumor-like mass in the colon)
  c. multiple poorly defined colonic filling defects simulating polyposis or a poorly prepared colon (adherent collections of viscid mucus)
  d. small, contracted, poorly functioning gallbladder (high incidence of gallstones)
  e. meconium ileus (bubbly or frothy pattern superimposed on numerous dilated loops of small bowel)
  f. fine granular pancreatic calcification (implies advanced pancreatic fibrosis associated with diabetes)

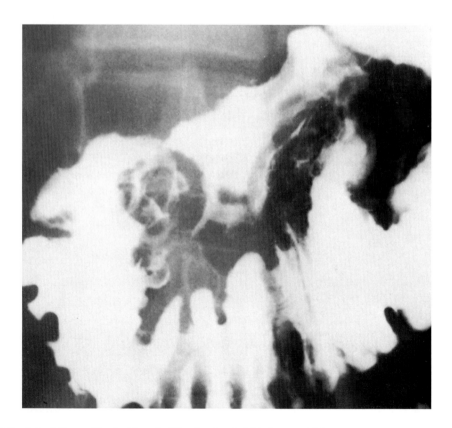

F I G U R E   3 4 - 1 3   Cystic fibrosis. The duodenal folds have a thick, coarse pattern.

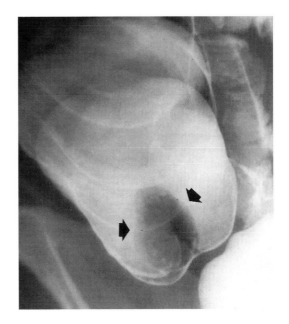

FIGURE 34-14
Cystic fibrosis. Tumor-like mass *(arrows)* in the cecum.

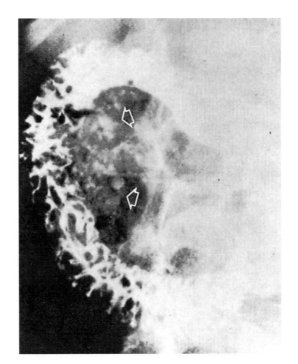

FIGURE 34-15
Cystic fibrosis. Finely granular calcifications *(arrows)*, primarily in the head of the pancreas. (From Ring EJ, Eaton SB, Ferrucci JT, et al. Differential diagnosis of pancreatic calcification. *AJR* 1973;117:446, with permission.)

Suggested Reading
Phelan MS, Fine DR, Zentler-Munro L, et al. Radiographic abnormalities of the duodenum in cystic fibrosis. *Clin Radiol* 1983;34:573.

Portal Vein Gas

KEY FACTS

- Presence of gas in the portal venous system usually has grave prognostic significance and is a sign of imminent death
- An exception is in relatively asymptomatic infants with umbilical vein catheters
- Major causes are necrotizing enterocolitis (children) and mesenteric arterial occlusion with bowel infarction (adults)
- Bubbles of gas embolizing to the portal vein are carried into the fine peripheral radicles in the liver by the centrifugal flow of portal venous blood (in contrast, gas in the biliary tree is found in larger, more centrally situated bile ducts)
- Characteristic radiographic appearance of radiating tubular lucencies branching from the porta hepatis to the edge of the liver
- Visualization of gas in the outermost 2 cm of the liver is considered to be presumptive evidence of portal vein gas

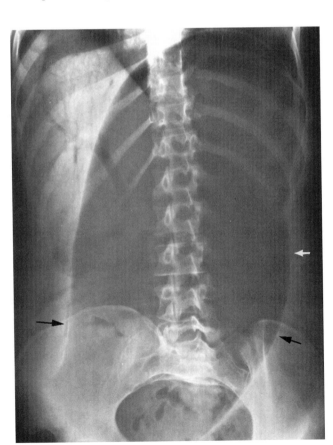

FIGURE 34-16

Portal vein gas. Branching radiolucencies in the right upper quadrant that extend almost to the edge of the liver. There is massive acute gastric dilatation with lucent streaks in the wall of the stomach *(arrows)*. (From Radin DR, Rosen RS, Halls JM. Acute gastric dilatation: a rare cause of portal vein gas. *AJR* 1987;148:279, with permission.)

FIGURE 34-17

Portal vein gas. CT scan shows extensive gas in the portal venous system in a patient with cirrhosis of the liver and marked ascites. (From Lund EC, Han SY, Holley HC, et al. Intestinal ischemia: comparison of plain radiographic and computed tomographic findings. *Radiographics* 1988;8:1083, with permission.)

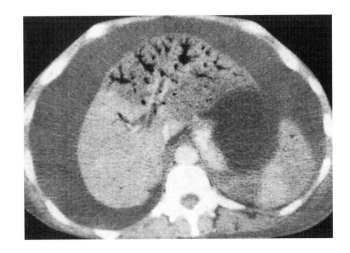

Suggested Reading

Rice RP, Thompson WM, Gedgaudas RK. The diagnosis and significance of extraluminal gas in the abdomen. *Radiol Clin North Am* 1982;20:819.

Gas in the Biliary Tree

KEY FACTS

- Related to disruption of the normal sphincter mechanism that prevents reflux of intestinal contents into both the bile and pancreatic ducts
- Most common cause is prior surgery, usually performed for biliary obstruction (primarily sphincterotomy)
- Inflammatory process can lead to gas in the biliary tree either by fistulization between the biliary system and the gastrointestinal tract (gallstone) or by anatomic distortion and resulting incompetence of the sphincter of Oddi (peptic ulcer disease, pancreatitis)
- Gas in the biliary tree is found in the larger, more centrally situated bile ducts (unlike portal vein gas, biliary gas is prevented from entering the finer radicles by the continuous centripetal flow of the secreted bile)

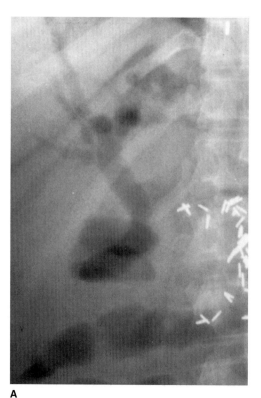 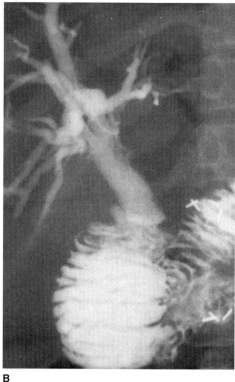

A   B

FIGURE 34-18   Gas in the biliary tree. **A:** Following a surgical procedure to relieve biliary obstruction, there is a large amount of gas within the bile ducts. **B:** Reflux of contrast material into the biliary system during an upper gastrointestinal series.

Suggested Reading

Rice RP, Thompson WM, Gedgaudas RK. The diagnosis and significance of extraluminal gas in the abdomen. *Radiol Clin North Am* 1982;20:819.

Nondiaphragmatic Hernias

PARADUODENAL HERNIA

KEY FACTS

- Represents more than half of all internal hernias (i.e., through a normal or abnormal aperture within the confines of the peritoneal cavity)
- Results from failure of the mesentery to fuse with the parietal peritoneum at the ligament of Treitz
- Three to four times more frequent on the left
- Bunched loops of small bowel that appear to be confined in a sac

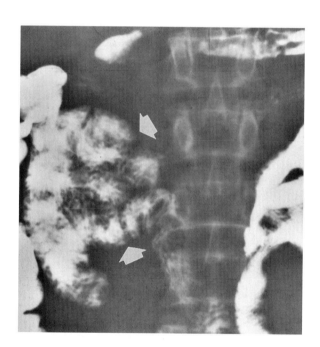

FIGURE 34-19
Right paraduodenal hernia. The jejunal loops are bunched together on the right side of the abdomen *(arrows)*, and the junction of the duodenum and jejunum has a low right paramedian position.

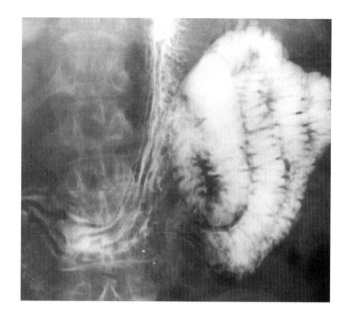

FIGURE 34-20
Left paraduodenal hernia. Small bowel loops are clustered in the left upper quadrant lateral to the fourth portion of the duodenum and the stomach.

Suggested Reading

Ghahremani GG. Internal abdominal hernias. *Surg Clin North Am* 1984;64:393.

LESSER SAC HERNIA

KEY FACTS

- Herniation through the foramen of Winslow that typically presents as an acute abdominal emergency (fatal intestinal strangulation unless prompt surgical relief)
- Collection of bowel and omentum in the left upper and mid-abdomen, displacing the stomach and transverse colon anteriorly
- Barium study or CT may show tapering of contrast-filled bowel pointing to the opening of the lesser sac

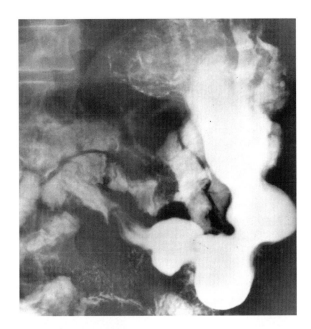

FIGURE 34-21

Lesser sac hernia (through the foramen of Winslow). Loops of small bowel are located in an abnormal position along the lesser curvature medial and posterior to the stomach.

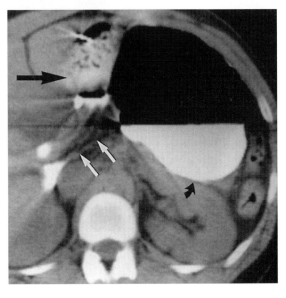

FIGURE 34-22

Lesser sac hernia. CT scan shows air and contrast material in a dilated cecum *(curved arrow)* posterior to the stomach *(large black arrow).* Note the beak-like contour of herniated bowel and stretched mesenteric vessels *(small white arrows)* at the foramen of Winslow. (From Wojtasek DA, Codner MA, Nowak EJ. CT diagnosis of cecal herniation through the foramen of Winslow. *Gastrointest Radiol* 1991;16:77, with permission.)

Suggested Reading

Wojtasek DA, Codner MA, Nowak EJ. CT diagnosis of cecal herniation through the foramen of Winslow. *Gastrointest Radiol* 1991;16:77.

INGUINAL HERNIA

KEY FACTS

- Classified as indirect or direct depending on its relation to the inferior epigastric vessels (indirect passes laterally; direct passes medially)
- Indirect hernias are more frequent, primarily occur in males, and account for 15% of intestinal obstructions (only neoplasms and adhesions are more common causes)
- On plain radiographs, gas-filled loops of bowel may be seen extending beyond the normal pelvic contour

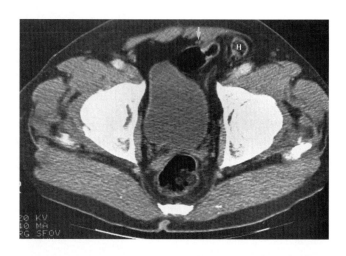

FIGURE 34-23
Indirect inguinal hernia. The neck of the hernia *(H)* is situated just lateral to the inferior epigastric vessels *(arrow)*. (From Wechsler RJ, Kurtz AB, Needleman L, et al. Cross-sectional imaging of abdominal wall hernias. *AJR* 1989;153:517, with permission.)

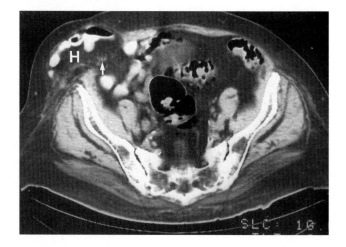

FIGURE 34-24
Direct inguinal hernia. The neck of the large hernia *(H)* is situated medial to the inferior epigastric vessels *(arrow)*. (From Wechsler RJ, Kurtz AB, Needleman L, et al. Cross-sectional imaging of abdominal wall hernias. *AJR* 1989;153:517, with permission.)

Suggested Reading
Wojasek DA, Codner MA, Nowak EJ. CT diagnosis of cecal herniation through the foramen of Winslow. *Gastrointest Radiol* 1991;16:77.

FEMORAL HERNIA

KEY FACTS

- Less common than inguinal hernias, but about ten times more prone to incarceration and strangulation
- More frequent in women
- On CT, a femoral hernia sac lies below and lateral to the pubic tubercle (whereas an inguinal hernia lies above and medial to the tubercle)

FIGURE 34-25
Femoral hernia. Fluid-filled loops of bowel *(asterisk)* lie along the course of the saphenous vein. (From Wechsler RJ, Kurtz AB, Needleman L, et al. Cross-sectional imaging of abdominal wall hernias. *AJR* 1989;153:517, with permission.)

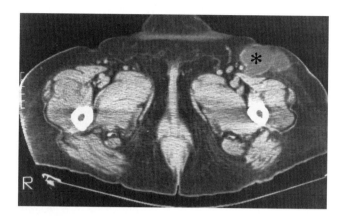

Suggested Reading

Wechsler RJ, Kurtz AB, Needleman L, et al. Cross-sectional imaging of abdominal wall hernias. *AJR* 1989;153:517.

OBTURATOR HERNIA

KEY FACTS

- Rare lesion that most frequently occurs on the right and in thin, older women
- Positive Howship-Romberg sign (pain along the inner aspect of the thigh to the knee or below, due to compression of the obturator nerve by the hernia contents)
- On CT, increased separation of the muscular bands of first the internal obturator muscle and then the external obturator muscle, before the hernia passes through the obturator canal and emerges between the pectineus and obturator externus muscles

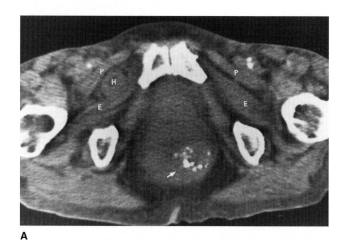

A

FIGURE 34-26
Obturator hernia. **A:** CT scan through the level of the symphysis shows a small bowel loop *(H)* herniated through the right obturator foramen between the pectineus **(P)** and external obturator **(E)** muscles. Of incidental note is calcification within a uterine fibroid *(arrow)*. **B:** CT scan illustrating the normal anatomy at the level of the symphysis pubis. (Meziane MA, Fishman EK, Siegelman SS. Computed tomography of obturator foramen hernia. *Gastrointest Radiol* 1983;8: 375.)

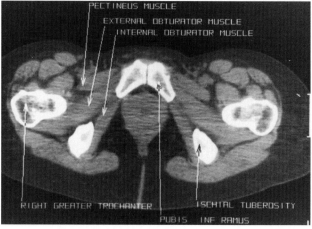

B

Suggested Reading

Meziane MA, Fishman EK, Siegelman SS. Computed tomographic diagnosis of obturator foramen hernia. *Gastrointest Radiol* 1983;8:375.

SCIATIC HERNIA

KEY FACTS

- Rare lesion that passes from the pelvis through the sciatic foramen into the buttocks (laterally into the subgluteal region)

FIGURE 34-27
Sciatic hernia. Recurrent rectal carcinoma *(asterisk)* herniating through the sciatic foramen lies behind the ischial spine deep to the gluteus maximus muscle *(G)*. (From Wechsler RJ, Kurtz AB, Needleman L, et al. Cross-sectional imaging of abdominal wall hernias. *AJR* 1989;153:517, with permission.)

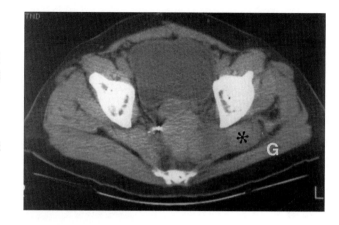

Suggested Reading

Wechsler RJ, Kurtz AB, Needleman L, et al. Cross-sectional imaging of abdominal wall hernias. *AJR* 1989;153:517.

HERNIATION THROUGH THE ANTERIOR ABDOMINAL WALL

KEY FACTS

- Umbilical, ventral, and postoperative incisional hernias
- Most are clinically apparent and imaging is used to demonstrate the nature of the herniated contents and to detect any bowel obstruction
- Incisional hernias that are not palpable (due to obesity or abdominal pain and distension) are easily detected on CT

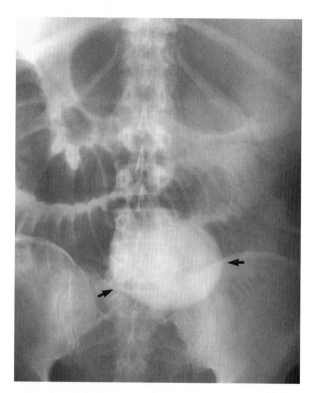

FIGURE 34-28
Strangulated umbilical hernia. Large soft-tissue mass *(arrows)* in the mid-abdomen and lower pelvis. The loops of small bowel proximal to the point of obstruction are dilated.

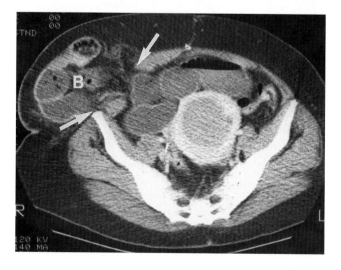

FIGURE 34-29
Obstructed incisional hernia. Dilated loops of bowel *(B)* extend into the abdominal wall through a defect in the region of the linea semilunaris *(arrows)*. This was the site of a previous surgical incision. (From Wechsler RJ, Kurtz AB, Needleman L, et al. Cross-sectional imaging of abdominal wall hernias. *AJR* 1989;153:517, with permission.)

Suggested Reading
Ghahremani GG, Jiminez MA, Rosenfeld M, et al. CT diagnosis of occult incisional hernias. *AJR* 1987;148:139.

OMPHALOCELE

KEY FACTS

- Protrusion of abdominal viscera into the base of the umbilical cord (with an associated defect in the abdominal wall)
- Represents persistence of normal fetal herniation with failure of complete withdrawal of the midgut from the umbilical cord during the tenth fetal week
- Complications include infection, rupture, and obstruction of bowel loops entering or exiting from the hernia sac

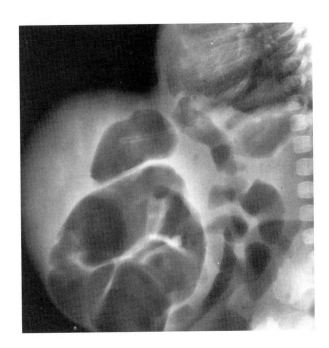

FIGURE 34-30
Omphalocele. Loops of gas-filled small bowel can be seen within the lesion.

Suggested Reading

Bair JH, Russ PD, Pretorius DH, et al. Fetal omphalocele and gastroschisis: a review of 24 cases. *AJR* 1986;147:1047.

SPIGELIAN HERNIA

KEY FACTS

• Lateral herniation through a spontaneous defect of the anterior abdominal wall along the linea semilunaris (lateral margin of the rectus muscle)

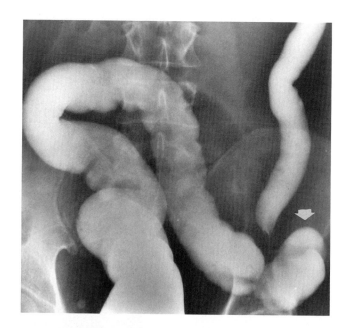

FIGURE 34-31
Spigelian hernia. Small bowel is trapped in the hernia sac *(arrow)*, which arises along the left semilunar line.

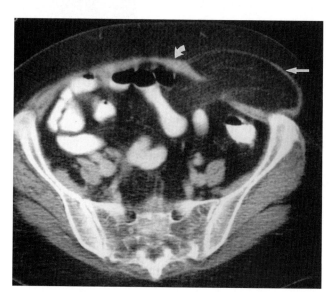

FIGURE 34-32
Spigelian hernia. Herniation of fat through a defect in the aponeurosis between the left rectus abdominis *(curved arrow)* and the aponeurosis of the left transversus abdominus and internal oblique muscles. The lateral margin of the hernia sac is the external oblique muscle and fascia *(straight arrow)*. (From Lee GHL,Cohen AJ. CT imaging of abdominal hernias. *AJR* 1993;161:1209, with permission.)

Suggested Reading
Lee GHL, Cohen AJ. CT imaging of abdominal hernias. *AJR* 1993;161:1209.

LUMBAR HERNIA

KEY FACTS

Occurs through either of two areas of relative weakness in the flank
  a. superior lumbar triangle (bounded by 12th rib superiorly, internal oblique muscle anteriorly, erector spinae muscle posteriorly)
  b. inferior lumbar triangle (bounded by external oblique muscle anteriorly, latissimus dorsi muscle posteriorly, iliac crest inferiorly)

- May be post-traumatic or spontaneous, and occurs most frequently on the left and in middle-aged men

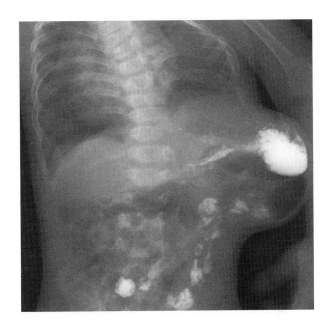

FIGURE 34-33
Lumbar hernia *(superior triangle)*. Note the multiple bony anomalies.

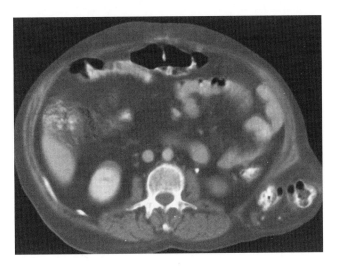

FIGURE 34-34
Lumbar hernia *(inferior triangle)*.

Suggested Reading
Faro SH, Racette CD, Lally JF, et al. Traumatic lumbar hernia: CT diagnosis. *AJR* 1990; 154:757.

Index